J
of PSYCHLER PATHOLOGY

Megan
Keep Psychly!
Dave Robinson
May '19

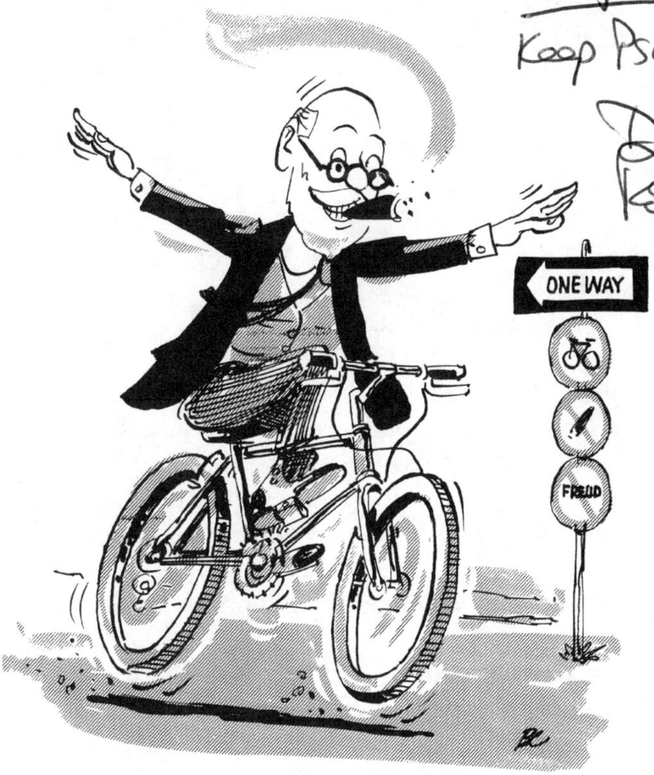

Edited by David J. Robinson, M.D.

Rapid Psychler Press

Suite 374
3560 Pine Grove Ave.
Port Huron, Michigan
USA 48060

Suite 203
1673 Richmond St.
London, Ontario
Canada N6G 2N3

Toll Free Phone 888-PSY-CHLE (888-779-2453)
Toll Free Fax 888-PSY-CHLR (888-779-2457)

Outside the U.S. & Canada — Phone 519-675-0610
Outside the U.S. & Canada — Fax 519-675-0610

website www.psychler.com
email rapid@psychler.com

ISBN 1-894328-01-9
Printed in the United States of America

First Edition, First Printing

All caricatures are purely fictitious. Any resemblance to real people, either living or deceased, is entirely coincidental (and unfortunate). The author assumes no responsibility for the consequences of diagnoses made, or treatment instituted, as a result of the contents of this book — such determinations should be made by qualified mental health professionals.

Dedication

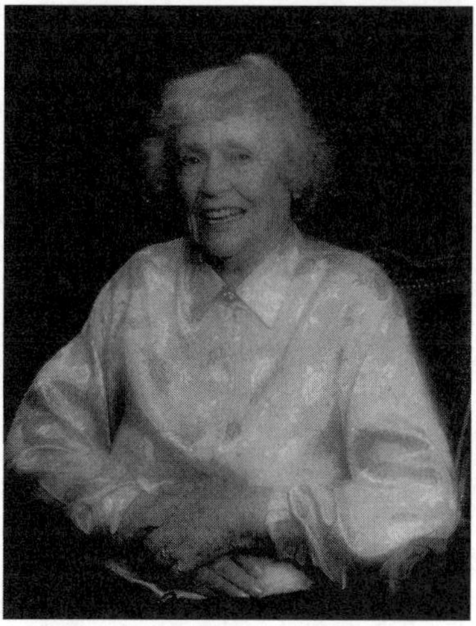

To my grandmother,

Frieda Sidona Brokop
1907 — 2001

Acknowledgments

I am indebted to the following individuals for their unfailing support and enthusiasm in assisting me with this project.

- **Monty & Lilly Robinson**
- **Brian Chapman**
- **Dr. Donna Robinson & Dr. Robert Bauer**
- **Brad Groshok & Susan McFarland**
- **Dean Avola**
- **Tom Kay**

Spoof Readers

- **Tom Norry, BSc.N.**
- **Sue Fletcher-Keron**
- **Noel Laporte, M.D.**
- **Martha Wilke, BSc.OT**
- **Marnie Desjardins, R.N.**
- **Vinay Lodha, M.D.**
- **Brenda Fuhrman, BSc.N., LL.B. & Emily Fuhrman**

A Special Thank You

- To all of the contributors who shared their ideas and allowed me to print their work.
- To the subscribers of the former *PsychoIllogical Bulletin* from which many of these articles were taken.
- To the readers of *Kick-in-the-Pants Therapy*. Your support and encouragement inspired me to publish another volume of caricatures and psychiatric satire.

Table of Contents

Author's Foreword

June, 1993 was a dangerous time for me. I had just finished my psychiatry residency and had a head full of ideas coupled with four years of suppressed creativity. I wrote a satirical article about ways of identifying people with personality disorders by their activities outside of a typical therapy session. I was hooked.

My initial publishing venture was called the *PsychoIllogical Bulletin*, the first edition of which was printed in 1994. I was fortunate to have many contributors and supporters in both the U.S. and Canada. My intention was to produce a humor periodical that contained short, punchy articles that would strike some people as at least mildly inappropriate. A good satire, by its very nature, has to hit home. I am blessed to have the time and talents of my godfather, Brian Chapman, to assist me in my publishing efforts. At this point time, he has drawn over 1000 illustrations and has been an outstanding collaborator. He often has the artwork completed months in advance of when I actually need it.

The *PsychoIllogical Bulletin* lasted for five years. During this time I changed my focus to writing humorous psychiatric textbooks that contained Brian's illustrations. I was no longer able to devote the resources to keeping the *Bulletin* going. The material from the first six volumes was published in book form as *Kick-in-the-Pants Therapy*. I continued to both write and receive satirical articles, and when I had enough material, I combined it with Volumes 7 — 10 to produce this book. I hope that the *Journal of Psychler Pathology* brings you as much joy as a reader as I had in putting it together.

Keep Psychling!

Dave Robinson

London, Ontario, Canada
March, 2003

Chapter 1. Academia

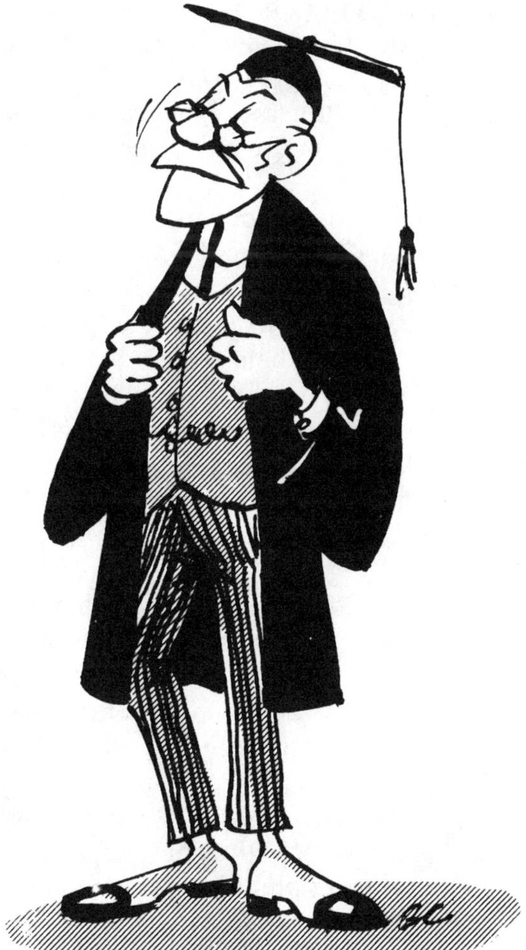

The Eminent Person Speaks:
A Nightmare of Grand Rounds

Sidney Hart, M.D.
Greenwich, Connecticut

Dr. George Awed: Good morning ladies and gentlemen, and welcome to the Grand Rounds for the Department of Psychiatry. We are indeed fortunate to have with us this morning the eminent psychiatrist *Dr. Hugo Kugelkopf*, who is currently Visiting Acting Professor Emeritus at the State University, where he occupies the prestigious Eames chair.

While I am sure that most of you are familiar with his distinguished career, and at the risk of being tiresome, let me review some of the high points of his professional life. Dr. Kugelkopf's brilliance was first apparent in medical school when he recognized, long before there was general acceptance of this, that the medial forebrain bundle is a highly significant neural structure. Unfortunately, his belief that "it is the ligament which holds the eyelids shut during a sneeze preventing the explosion of the brain through the eye sockets," has not stood the test of time.

Undaunted by this disappointment, Kugelkopf proceeded through a residency in psychiatry and pursued analytic training as a post-graduate. Renowned as a defender of the faith and a strict "constructionist" in interpreting analytic principles, he is reported not to have uttered one word in the years 1952, 1959, and 1960. This is actually an overstatement. Studebaker has noted that in 1959, while visiting his tailor, Kugelkopf broke the silence when he was unable to resist a little joke; when his tailor pinned his scrotum to the inseam of his pants, Kugelkopf remarked ironically, "Ginsberg, are you here to alter me or my pants?"

He never forgave himself this violation of technique, and, due to the acute shortage of parameters that year following the ban on their importation, was unable to introduce one to Ginsberg, terminating their relationship.

In 1960, his analytic practice suffered a sudden reversal as patient after patient left his consulting room in tears with the complaint "the material is too painful." In a subsequent letter to Flyss, the Norwegian analyst, Kugelkopf bemoaned the experience, "I had just reupholstered the analytic couch with my own blend of polyester and copper. How was I to know that this fabric could generate 400 volts between two sweaty palms?"

Dr Kugelkopf recognized the fact that neuroleptics would completely alter the practice of psychiatry in the 1960's and he devoted himself to research in the field for the next decade. His use of phenothiazines in the treatment of exhibitionism is a classic. Kugelkopf capitalized on the side effects of these drugs and induced such horrifying and unsightly tardive dyskinesias that his patients were too ashamed to bare their faces, let alone their nether parts, in public.

Staying abreast of the changes in the field, Kugelkopf soon found himself deeply involved in Community Psychiatry. An expert on the use of surrogate therapists and indigenous healers, he envisioned a true therapeutic community in which every person would perform therapy for every other person. Not satisfied with the exclusive use of hairdressers and bartenders — they were too limited — he trained supermarket check-out girls in Kinesiology and had them make dynamic interpretations to the shoppers who fumbled with their change as it was poured over the conveyor in front of them.

The Human Potential Movement had a great appeal to the doctor, and he saw potential that others failed to perceive.

His own technique of nude underwater encounter groups, or, **Naqueous Therapy**, was an immediate success in California and Florida, though less so in Arizona. Of this therapy Kugelkopf is reported to have said, "it changed my wife."

But it is his current work for which his greatest accolades have been reserved. The use of behavioral techniques and biofeedback appealed to him immensely. They completely circumvent the murky and treacherous waters of the unconscious, require less time and money, allow for the immediate confrontation of transference resistances, and ultimately leave the patient in complete control of his fate. This, he thought, was the truest form of self help, and led to the coining of the term **Behaviorself Therapy**.

Ladies and Gentlemen, it is with great pleasure I present to you Dr. Hugo Kugelkopf.

Dr. Hugo Kugelkopf: Thank you for your generous introduction, Dr. Todd, and say hello to your charming wife for me when you get home. I am indeed pleased to be here this morning to discuss past and future developments in the field. As Freud said to Jung one day as they approached Bergasse 19, "Carl, after a hot corned beef sandwich, I always like a nice glass of tea."

I am indebted to Joe Namath for that story which he related to me over a splendid dinner at Steve and Edie's last month when we were planning the J. Robert Oppenheimer Memorial Scholarship Rock Concert featuring "Little Eddie and the Mammary Glands."

Freud and Jung had a falling out, as you know, because Freud was convinced that Jung both wished him dead and had a revolting taste in ties. Jung was an incorrigible practical joker and Freud often misinterpreted this trickery as treachery. Once, Jung had managed to tie Ernest Jones' shoelaces together when he, Jones, Freud, and Tyco Brahe were at the Paris Opera and Jones went down the Grand Staircase like Gene Kelly in *An American in Paris* to the applause and wonderment of Paris society. Another time, Jung managed to slip Freud an exploding cigar with a charge so powerful that when it detonated it propelled Freud's glasses across the room nearly wounding Fleiss, who at the time was lost in a reverie which carelessly had been left hanging between the fireplace and an end table.

But I am digressing. I am here to inform you not regale you with anecdotes. But, just the other day, Herbert Von Karajan was telling me and Ann Margaret about the time that he and Rudolf Serkin — whoops! There I go again!

Please understand that anecdotalism is an affliction of eminent persons. It becomes even worse when one graduates from eminence to greatness. Great persons sneak almost exclusively in to the anecdotal form. Ah! I see some of the young people in the audience are snickering. Snickering! Well, my eminence is a fact that your laughter cannot erase! I am a member of the Academy, the Association, the Board, the Council, the Department, the Institute, the Society, and the Hertz Number One Club!

I wish to move now to the issue of treatment. Many years ago I made the observation that snails are very slow, even sluggish creatures proceeding tediously towards their goal — usually a slime pile or a dead fish. "Well", you say, "who would be in a hurry to get there?" But that is precisely where genius differs from the ordinary person. It occurred to me that, like the snail, the depressed person is also sluggish and tedious, especially when doing a polka or the *cha cha*. "Perhaps the snail can teach us something about depression," I said to myself, as I was much ignored in the early years of my career. There were many advantages to working with these animals. They were cheap, often being given away free with guppies at pet stores; they were easy to keep and feed; they didn't bite or give an electric shock and, after a day's work, they made a fine snack when cooked up with a little butter and garlic and served with a well-chilled Puligny-Montrachet. My predicament, having training in neither chemistry nor physiology, was how to begin to study my hypothesis. Fortunately, those were the days when there was lots of money available for research and I received many grants to aid me in my efforts to frame the problem, and an approach to it. That I failed to produce either had little effect upon my funding for almost twenty years. Eventually, I grew tired of the project and turned to more clinical issues.

I moved to Chicago at about that time, where the great Franz Alexander was espousing a technique of psychotherapy (**The Corrective Emotional Experience**) which attempted to correct the psychic traumas inflicted upon children by their relentlessly stupid and bungling parents. These "introjected parental imagos" (or "amigos" in Esperanto) continued to torment their possessors like unruly tenants in a Co-op. Now, I know some of you are skeptical about this concept of introjection, but let me assure you that children are capable of remarkable acts of internalization — that which an adult would never dream possible. For example, when I was a boy, I used to eat onions the way other kids ate apples, yet today if you so much as show me a shallot, I get heartburn like you wouldn't believe!

Building upon my conceptualizations, I devised a variant of Alexander's technique which I call **The Corrective Immotional Experience**. In this treatment, when a patient does not accept an interpretation, he is tied to the couch and left over night. I have found, since employing this simple strategy, that most of my patients have gained insight more rapidly and aside from a curious but dreadful fear of being asked to play Joan of Arc at parties, have not substituted new symptoms in place of the old.

Currently, I am experimenting with a new twist based on the work of Otto Kernberg which I call **Object Deletions Theory**. With this tactic, if a patient quarrels about the accuracy of a clarification or confrontation, his shoes are taken away from him. This is remarkably effective, particularly on snowy days, and you can be certain the patient thinks twice before being disagreeable again!

I can see my time is almost up, but there are several points I'd like to make before closing, especially for the young therapists and resident physicians in the audience.

1. Always introduce yourself to your patient. This is particularly important for the patient with a split personality so he can be sure which of the two of the three of you in the room, is/are him.

2. There are only three times when you should shake a patient's hand: at the end of the first meeting; at the end of the last meeting; and when the patient wishes to slip you a little something extra for a job well done.

3. Don't sit at your desk during therapy sessions. It puts a barrier between you and the patient, making you seem remote and imperious; and if you happen to doze off, you could give your head a terrible knock on a sharp corner or drawer handle.

4. Finally, never give advice to patients. Sell it to them.

Thank you very much.

Political Solutions to Classroom Problems:

Avoiding Questions You Can't or Don't Want to Answer

Steven J. Kirsh, Ph.D.
Geneseo, New York

During a lecture, professors are occasionally forced to respond to questions for which they simply don't know the answer. Because these questions are distracting, tangential, strange or just plain wacky, this article lists the ten most useful dodges for avoiding having to provide an answer.

Response # 10

"Great question! You've shown a keen understanding of the problem. What led you to think of that question?"

Rationale: Use this response if you don't have a clue about the answer but don't want to look stupid. By forcing the student to tell you the derivation of the question, you might get the information you need to reply. If the student doesn't ante up, say that his or her allotment of one question was used up and then move on.

Response # 9

"Wow, what an advanced question. Unfortunately that one's beyond the scope of this course. You'll have to save it for the next semester."

Rationale: By default, if you can't answer the question, it has to be beyond the level of the course. By emphasizing the sophistication of the question, you can deflect attention from your ignorance by building the esteem of the student.

Response # 8

"You know how sometimes during a test you forget the answer, but it pops into your mind as soon as you leave the room? That's what's happening to me right now."

Rationale: This response helps you save face by indicating you once knew the answer, even if you never did. By relating to common exam experiences, you come across as pretty hip.

Response # 7

"Does anyone in the class know the answer?"

Rationale: This deflects responsibility for the errant questioner onto the class instead of you. If no one knows the answer, make it an assignment to be handed in. Very soon the perpetrator will get silenced.

Response # 6

Compose an answer, but quote recent or obscure authorities. For example, "According to Clinton. . ." or "Recent findings suggest that . . ."

Rationale: This answer makes you appear as if you keep up on the literature in your field. If you get called on this, say that you are a reviewer for a prestigious journal and have access to drafts of future articles.

Response # 5

"I don't know."

Rationale: This response humanizes even the most extra-terrestrial-looking faculty member. It should be used cautiously because it erodes your reputation as the local expert. If you in turn use the question posed in class on a future exam, you must be prepared to give full marks for this answer.

Response # 4

"I'm not completely sure, but I think. . ."

Rationale: By hedging your reply, you at least give the appearance of having a functioning coconut on your shoulders. Besides, can we ever really know anything for certain?

Response # 3

"I'd love to respond to that question, but there isn't enough time if we are to cover the material that's going to be on the next exam."

Rationale: This allows you to maintain your dignity and not lie to your students. You didn't say you'd *answer* the question, just *respond* to it. Simply put, this means that you don't have time to tell your students that you don't know the answer. Your evaluations will soar by giving the indication you actually intend to teach (or even just mention) something that might be on the exam.

Response # 2

"That's a very difficult question to answer. . . but I happen to know a lot about this area. . ." Then, give an obsessively-detailed overly-inclusive answer to the question.

Rationale: When you know the answer, spare no effort to call attention to your expertise, even if you learned it by watching CNN. Responses of this nature will act as negative reinforcement for future challenges to your knowledge.

Response # 1

Make the gesture of asking if there are any questions, but prevent any from being asked by immediately launching on to a completely different topic. Remind the class about your office hours if something does come up.
Rationale: This tangential tactic preempts pesky questions.

By the time one of the little ingrates comes up with something, he or she won't ask it because you'll have moved onto more fertile (or fertilized) areas. If you are tracked down in your office, at least you won't have an audience to attest to your mental lapses.

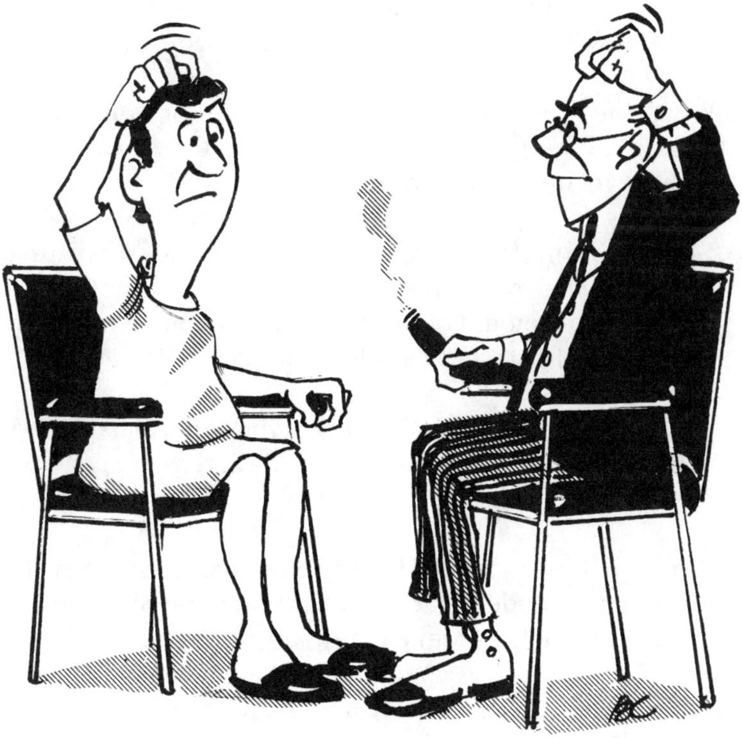

The Top Ten Signs (S.D. 2) You've Been Doing Too Much Research

Carolyn Sullins, M.S.
Champaign, Illinois

1. Someone calling for an employment reference asks how reliable your employee was, and you answer in terms of Pearson's Product Moment or Rulon's Formula.

2. When the toaster sets off the smoke detector, you scream, "That's a Type-I error! Honey, can you please lower the alpha level on that damn thing!"

3. You start formulating regression equations for predicting your own state of neurosis, with beta weights for the predictors of amount of sleep, amount of homework, daily intake of caffeine, and days left until qualifying exams.

4. You see "Box O' Clusters" cereal in the supermarket, and wonder how that compares to multi-dimensional scaling cereal.

5. While on the same shopping trip, you figure out the mean, median and mode of the products you're buying — after discarding the least and most expensive items.

6. When your friends accuse you of being neurotic, you ask them what actuarial evidence they have for this assertion.

7. If the answer to the above question is, "Everybody just knows you're neurotic," you point out the methodological limitations of inter-rater reliability.

8. If your friends still insist that you're neurotic, you point out the lack of ecological validity and generalizability in this statement. After all, they have only observed your neurosis in terms of your academic life, which doesn't necessarily generalize to other aspects of your so-called life.

9. You then realize you have no other aspect to your life, but statistically, neither do most people.

10. You take the term "standard deviant" as a compliment.

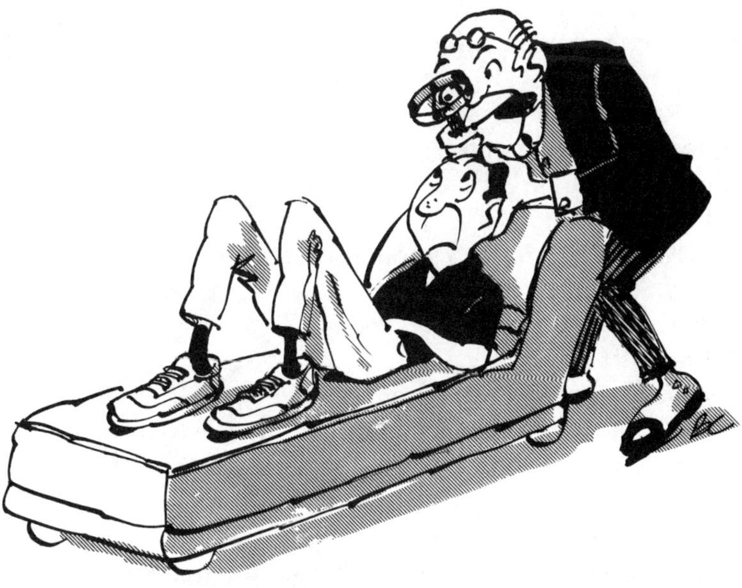

Faculty Members Drive Saturns, Administrators Drive You Crazy

Michael F. Shaughnessy, Ph.D.
Portales, New Mexico

This article examines the communication difficulties between administration and faculty members. Actual dialogue between these time-honored opponents is presented using the following framework:

- What is actually said by the faculty member
- The distorted "meta-message" perceived by the administrator
- The reply given by the administrator

Faculty Member Says. . .
"I need a new computer to perform various detailed statistical analyses on my data."
Administrator Hears. . .
My eight-year old Radio Shack Special can only play the demo version of Space Ranger. I want to be able to play more interesting games with enhanced sounds and first-person graphics.
Administrator Says. . .
"Those 5¼ inch discs are practically new! Besides, first there was RAM, then ROM, and I'm waiting for RUM to be released. Then I'll spring for an upgrade."

Faculty Member Says. . .
"We can't get anyone to cover the summer course that has been scheduled for the 7:00 a.m. time slot."
Administrator Hears. . .
I see where this is going. There is nobody around to get the coffee made that early in the morning. Next there will be a request to have donuts delivered by the campus police.

Administrator Says. . .
"Well, you only teach a few hours a day — does it really matter which hours they are?"

Faculty Member Says. . .
"Dr. Shaughnessy is leaving at the end of the semester. Unless he is replaced, we will all have more than our allotted share of teaching assignments."
Administrator Hears. . .
This opportunist is trying to get on a Search Committee to get time away from work and eat shrimp at the university's expense. Nipping this in the bud is a cost-cutting strategy that I could be credited with.
Administrator Says. . .
"Why not just get a list of the alumni printed on 3" x 5" index cards, shuffle them and pick a replacement?"

Faculty Member Says. . .
"I need more funding for my research project."
Administrator Hears. . .
This whiner wants me to solve his problems. If I throw enough bureaucracy in his face, he'll go away.
Administrator Says. . .
"That will have to go through the Academic Council, the Dean's Committee, the Planning and Analysis Office and the Clandestine Brotherhood of Institutional Research Saboteurs. Let me know when you've spoken with each of them."

Faculty Member Says. . .
"We have a student who needs only one course to graduate. Unfortunately, it isn't offered this semester."
Administrator Hears. . .
The buck doesn't even slow down here, dummy. What'll I do next — deny, defer, or destroy? What would Dilbert do?
Administrator Says. . .
"Bring me the head of the student advisor!"

The Institute for Motivated Behavior

Joel Kirschbaum, Ph.D.
Hillsborough, New Jersey

The Institute for Motivated Behavior was developed to be an academic version of the guys from Bud Light® — we are here to help! It has come to our attention that there are retention problems concerning low-level underpaid faculty in today's teaching centers. We're not sure if this refers to classic anal retention or simply getting people to stick around. While we await clarification on this issue, we will solve the second problem first.

What is it that highly qualified people can get from a university that they can't get anywhere else? It's not money, it's not frustration, and it's not even preferred parking. Time to think outside the box — what are you going to do?

It is a title! People will work for years doing fruitless research, teaching the same class to bored undergrads, and toiling in the same institutional atmosphere all for the chance to get an improved title. This intangible designation appears to be worth the indignity of having one's life's work laid before a committee of hypocritical and hypercritical peers.

Apparently the whole process is worth it. With an improved title, you get a nice certificate, new business cards, new stationery, individualized envelopes, and lots of satisfaction in supplying personal information on official forms. The solution to the problem is to have more titles! Why just have a couple of hurdles when you can keep people hopping for more every couple months. All that is needed is a list of adjectives, a big stack of business cards, and a laser printer. Now to solve the first problem. . .

Examples of Additional Titles Granted Between Two Present Positions Within an Academic Hierarchy

Associate Professor

Most Excellent Assistant Professor
Adjacent Assistant Professor
Sub-Assistant Professor
Subordinate Assistant Professor
Inordinate Assistant Professor
Semi-Assistant Professor
Demi-Assistant Professor
Supplemental Assistant Professor
Deputy Assistant Professor
Auxiliary Assistant Professor
Ancillary Assistant Professor
Senior Assistant Professor
Intermediate Assistant Professor
Junior Assistant Professor
Executive Assistant Professor
Exalted Assistant Professor
Ascended Assistant Professor
Supra-Assistant Professor
Percolated Assistant Professor
Elevated Assistant Professor
Escalated Assistant Professor
Enhanced Assistant Professor
Increased Assistant Professor
Heightened Assistant Professor
Special Assistant Professor
General Assistant Professor
Major Assistant Professor
Minor Assistant Professor

Assistant Professor

The Title-to-Text Word-Count Ratio of a Published Journal Article and the Narcissistic Illusion of Accomplishment by its Author: A New Measure of Solipsistic Ego-Inflation

Steven J. Gilbert, Ph.D.
SUNY at Oneonta, New York

Of the million journal articles published yearly (Broad, 1988), only mine contains more words in the title (24)[1] than in its text (23)!

References

Broad, W.J.
Science Can't Keep up With the Flood of New Journals
The New York Times, pp C1-2, February 16, 1988

[1] "Text" word count is exclusive of reference citations, footnotes and the contents of the *References* section.

text/title ratio = 23/24 = 0.958

Ten Ways to P*** off a Psychology Graduate Student

Carolyn Sullins, M.S.
Champaign, Illinois

- Say . . . are you analyzing what I'm saying right now?
- I have this friend who . . . (insert twenty minutes of rambling dialogue describing the friend's eccentric habits) . . . would you diagnose her with Maniac-Depression or what?
- So, you're going to be paid $100/hour just to have people tell you about their problems? Must be nice!
- I've heard that most people become therapists because they're trying to figure out what's wrong with them. Is that true for you?
- Dr. Laura Schlessinger is **great**. Are you going to be like her?
- I don't need a therapist, I have you as my friend/daughter/ etc.
- You've been in school for HOW long?
- I have a friend who got his B.A. the same time you got yours, and now he makes 80K a year.
- I'll be your first patient *after* you graduate.
- What! You've got personal problems? But you're a therapist, don't you know how to fix them yourself?

Schedule of a Typical Professional Program for Psychiatrists

(with Approved CME Credits)

Morning Session

9:00 — 9:05	Opening Remarks
9:05 — 9:15	Introductions
9:15 — 9:30	Discussion of opening remarks and introductions
10:00 — 12:00	Coffee break

Afternoon Session

12:00 — 3:00	Lunch
3:00 — 4:00	Discussion of coffee break and lunch
4:00 — 5:00	Adjournment
5:00 — 5:30	Discussion of Adjournment

Lewis H. Richmond, M.D.
San Antonio, Texas

How to Read Clinical Journals:

Sounding Like You've Read the Literature When You Haven't Read a Thing

Donald A. Redelmeier, M.D. Miriam Shuchman, M.D., & Steven L. Shumak, M.D.

Many clinicians do not regularly read journals, can't remember the details or confound the data with misinformation. Consider the following situations:
(a) You're in clinic, prescribing a lipid-lowering medication for a patient, and your medical student inquires about research suggesting the drug is associated with violent injury. How do you respond?
(b) You're on rounds when a colleague asks about a study linking computers to cancer. Some house staff are listening. How do you respond? In this article we outline methods for handling these types of situations. Our goal is to present effective strategies for practitioners to use when they need to pretend they've been keeping up with the medical journals. As with previous articles in this series, the guidelines we offer constitute "applied common sense" and are relevant to diverse clinical settings. The intent is to help you to masquerade as someone who regularly reads the literature.

1. Distract the Questioner

Canny physicians learn to cultivate a frantic atmosphere so that lesser issues can be side-stepped. For example, when asked "Did you see the latest report in *CMAJ* on bypass surgery?", try answering with "Oops, I left my laptop computer in the library after downloading a search!" This eliminates the risk of saying the wrong thing while simultaneously conveying a scholarly image. If sufficiently clever, this type of distraction gets stronger with repetition. Consider, for example, the rejoinder "That's the third time today I've left it behind!" Seems more convincing, doesn't it? Diverting the questioner is fun and easy. Sometimes we favour a pompous approach, such as "I'll answer that in a moment, but first let me talk about a recent triumph of mine." The secret here is to be long-winded rather than exciting. Alternatively, sometimes we adopt a more emotional approach by stealing lines from Marcus Welby. A favourite is: "This is not an easy topic for me. I remember an earlier patient. . ." Let your imagination run wild, and even a swift questioner can't catch you.

2. Redirect the Conversation

What if you don't want to kill the conversation? Have no fear, because less evasive strategies can also convey a scholarly image when you're clueless. Consider the following 2 lines: "I remember serving as a reviewer for that article a year ago for *CMAJ*. I recommended acceptance but can't remember the details right now." Notice the brilliance. You assert your scientific authority. You justify any lapses of memory. Moreover, you can't be faulted no matter where it was published. Redirection can follow any orientation of the compass. Try being grandiose, such as: "I know of other work by a high-profile colleague that will entirely change the field; however, I'm not allowed to talk about it yet." Try being self-deprecating, as in "I'd love to answer that but my colleague Dr. X would get offended because she considers herself the authority." Try being obsequious, as in "I think Dr. X said it best the other day; perhaps I can find her for you." Any of these will work fine.

3. Hog the High Road

Only the mediocre are always at their best and always polite. Thus, the occasional combative response is fine. Self-righteousness works well. Try "That's exactly the type of terrible science that wastes public dollars and should never have been supported when other, more important issues deserve attention." Notice how bruising this will be to the earnest questioner. In addition, it allows you to exploit any other current tragedy for your own personal gain. Styles of intimidation vary by personality and generally work better in Canada than the US. Some prefer methodologic rebuffs such as "That study was seriously flawed by a small sample that does not apply to my patient." Others prefer a clandestine style, as in "There's stuff you don't know that I can't tell you." Still others prefer an ad-hominem approach, as in "Those scientists are only interested in advancing their careers and not in improving the health of my patient." All these lines contain no information, cannot be falsified and fully terminate discussion.

4. Waffle Like a Pro

Doctors frequently take a dim view of politicians and thereby miss opportunities to learn from masters of rhetoric. Watch a member of parliament demonstrate lines such as "Well, the answer to that question really depends on your perspective. Sure, there are going to be some people who will be better off. But there are also going to be some who aren't. There may be other complications as well. It's difficult to predict. And there are other priorities too." Admire how such comments are so lengthy and so vacuous.

Indeed, physicians receive more professional training than politicians and thereby should be capable of even more elaborate rhetoric. Try the orthodox line, "The results are quite intriguing; still, I'd like to see these findings confirmed by other groups before I commit myself." Or the cosmic line, "It's a big issue that we don't have time for now. It's so big and important that I want to avoid giving you a fast response." Or the elitist line, "I used to believe I knew the answer to that question, but now I'm not so sure."

Summary

Keeping up with the literature is essential for being a leader in medicine. Yet who has the time? We suggest, therefore, that good pretending is an essential clinical skill that should be taught in medical school, practiced during patient care and honed at CME courses. Ironically, faking your way through the literature may also be a near-optimal use of time given that research is rarely definitive. Most studies won't stand the test of time, and realizing this encourages rational clinicians to ignore them all.

Our article has offered 4 guidelines for bluffing when asked factual questions about the medical literature. We know that the articles are difficult to read and easy to forget. So, we encourage you to use our guidelines when commenting on them. To consolidate your understanding, try also to write a letter to the editor about an article you've not seen. In addition, recognize that ongoing research is needed because standards for bluffing may change as the field of evidence-based medicine evolves.

David Sackett, Gordon Guyatt, Deborah Cook and David Naylor provided helpful points on early drafts, but we didn't listen.

No granting agency made the mistake of funding this work.

We bluffed our way past the editors by claiming no financial conflict of interest.

Reprinted with permission of the Canadian Medical Association Journal.
This article was originally published in:
CMAJ • DEC. 15, 1998; 159 (12) 1488 — 1489

How to Read Clinical Journals:

How to React When Your Colleagues Haven't Read a Thing

Steven L. Shumak, M.D., and Donald A. Redelmeir, M.D.

Abstract

Physicians receive little instruction on how to interact with colleagues, and even less guidance on what to do when their colleagues are poorly informed. Eight techniques are presented here that may be of use in dealing with colleagues who have clearly not read the literature and are unable to maintain the facade that they have. If employed properly and used judiciously, these techniques may help avoid embarrassment for all and may also improve the exchange of valuable information between professionals.

Earlier in this series we reviewed the important topic of how to read medical journals, including the specific task of "sounding like you've read the literature when you haven't read a thing." Consider the following scenario. During rounds with your colleague, you see a hypertensive patient suffering from a transient ischemic attack due to atrial fibrillation. Your colleague comments that anticoagulation is not indicated in this patient given its minimal efficacy for preventing cardioembolic events. Do you respond by saying, "OK," and then finish rounds by yourself that night after supper? Or do you reply with, "Yes. And by the way, how's that new position looking?" knowing full well that this position is at a premier teaching hospital where the house staff make the real decisions. Or perhaps, "No. Stay away from my patient. Don't make me call security." In this article, we suggest some diplomatic methods for handling this type of situation. Some physicians are terrific at dealing with patients but pathetic at dealing with other physicians. Our goal is to present effective strategies for busy practitioners to use when they need to talk with colleagues who are out of date or out of line. As with previous articles in this series, these guidelines constitute "applied common sense," are relevant to diverse clinical settings, and are especially valuable when interacting with trainees. Our methods emphasize the prevention of embarrassment, the preservation of collegiality and the teaching of a thing or two. As realists, though, we'll settle for 2 of 3.

1. Assume Responsibility For Their Mistake

Turning the tables is an easy and kind way of dealing with this problem. Suppose your colleague says, "Screening mammography in women over the age of 50 is a waste of time and resources." You might respond with, "It's my fault for not giving rounds about this. Screening in this situation is certainly important. I guess I should have worked harder to review things with everybody." Alternatively, if you have given rounds on just that point and now need to repeat that lesson, you should try, "I told you that, didn't I? But you know, I was wrong. Turns out that there's now strong evidence showing. . ." Turning the tables in this way requires a certain degree of confidence and may not be suitable for the more diffident among us. Also, when using this technique, there is a danger that your reputation could get somewhat tarnished. It's yet another example of where you must sacrifice yourself in the hope of achieving better patient outcomes.

2. Pretend You Misheard

This is a safe technique that maintains your intellectual stature. Anyone can use it, although it helps to have cultivated a reputation for having worked through medical school as a jackhammer operator. Consider the following hypothetical exchange. Your colleague says, "Well, one thing's for sure. There's hardly any role for cholesterol reduction after a myocardial infarction." You say, "Absolutely. Well put. A very *hearty* role indeed. What with all the studies showing the benefit of cholesterol reduction, it's surprising that statins aren't being put in the drinking water. Which one would you recommend I use?" Note the skill displayed here. First, you've turned the ignorance around and have actually complimented your colleague for bringing up such an important issue. Second, you've informed him about the current evidence and even alluded to the best treatment with statins. Third, you've slipped in a clever pun to help maintain good spirits for all. Well done! Of course, this approach can lead to problems if overused. Consider this exchange. Your colleague says, "Those vitamin fanatics! Now they say that all pregnant women should take folate." You reply, "You're right. Vitamins are *fantastic*. I'm finding more and more uses for them." Your colleague says, "As a friend, I have to say that I'm worried about your hearing." You (continuing the facade) respond, "Well, it's the year 2000 and I don't think anyone will mind if I wear an earring!"

3. Blame Someone or Something Else

With the proliferation of panels, guidelines and the like, it is now easy to find a scapegoat for the mistakes of a colleague. So, when your colleague asserts that "there's nothing to be gained by striving for improved glucose control in diabetic patients," you could respond with, "You know, I can see why you're confused. One panel says this, another says that. And another says this *and* that. What we need is an expert panel to guide the experts!" This approach may be especially valuable if you can trace the fault back to medical school, as with the response, "Actually, you're wrong. But it's not your fault. It's that damn new curriculum!" This technique can be extended to essentially any area. And even if your colleague's medical school curriculum did cover the problem, who cares? He or she is not going to point that out. We should also note explicitly that a shared rant (and it will be shared — your colleagues will definitely nod in agreement and possibly slam their fists down on a convenient surface) has its own benefits in collegial bonding. Given the endless vogue of curriculum renewal, this technique will have widespread utility and enduring relevance.

4. Pretend You Think They're Joking

This approach is quite simple and really needs no explanation. And, since everyone in the medical profession believes that they have a better than average sense of humour, there's nobody you can't use it on. Once more, a simple example suffices. Your colleague says, "Well, I really don't think that there's much to be gained by employing the 'Ottawa' ankle rules." You (beginning to chuckle) respond, "Yeah. What a laugh. Very funny. I know what you mean. We can't trust too much of anything that comes out of the nation's capital." It is important to understand, however, that the use of humour requires talent. Its use should be reserved for those professionals who can still tell a joke, yet remain politically correct. Of course, if you are truly gifted at being funny, you should leave medical practice immediately and make a much greater contribution to human welfare through the entertainment industry. And more money too.

5. Give Permission for Error

This technique is especially useful when you are dumbstruck by a colleague's approach, or lack thereof. So, when your usually sharp colleague says, "I'm not aware of any evidence to suggest that bedridden patients should receive deep vein thrombosis prophylaxis," you respond with, "Actually, there is. But, what with so many things to learn, memorize, relearn and then re-memorize as new developments come forth, it's impossible to keep on top of everything." Unlike some approaches reviewed in this article, this technique has the merit of being honest and is, therefore, especially useful if you have a conscience.

6. Find The One In A Million Case Where They're Right and Segue Back to Reality

This approach is best illustrated by an example. Suppose your colleague is considering that Mr. Jones, a 75-year-old man who's never been outside Sudbury, has hematuria due to schistosomiasis. You might respond with "I see what you're getting at. Always thinking, aren't you? You must have seen that case report in the Journal of 'X' " (with "X" being something you're sure he doesn't know exists and, in fact, may *not* exist). "Well, let's keep that in mind, but you know his prostate was huge on digital rectal. . ." This technique may be most suitable, and almost obligatory, for trainees. Consider the following encounter regarding an otherwise well 50-year-old woman, Ms. Smith, who has classic carpal tunnel syndrome. A student says, "I think that we really must rule out acromegaly. Ms. Smith, do you have headaches, visual changes, oily skin?" You say, "I told you, Ms. Smith, these students are getting more and more clever. And it's great to see that they keep an open mind. I guess if you're like me and have seen hundreds of cases, you tend to close your mind a bit and focus on the common."

7. Make The Mistake Part of a Raging Academic Debate

Despite its designation, use of this tactic is not restricted to academic centers. Consider the following example. Your colleague asks, "Do you know any good neurosurgeons? I just saw a fellow with a right carotid bruit and a 30% right internal carotid stenosis." You (using technique 5) respond with, "That's a 'toughie.' There's been so much written about therapy for cerebrovascular disease that it's hard to know what's best. Still, I'm pretty confident that nothing specific is needed, certainly not an operation." Colleague (resisting) says, "You're telling me he doesn't need surgery?" You (initiating technique 7) reply, "You've stumbled into the vortex of controversy. You can't pick up a journal without coming across this debate. People can get pretty heated talking about it, so be careful. I wouldn't operate unless it's symptomatic, and then only if the stenosis is greater than 70%."

8. Rejoice In Finding An Ally Against Nature's Absurdity

Who has not been chagrined at the counterintuitive aspects of medicine? Who has not been disappointed when some hard-learned physiologic understanding becomes a liability? The canny clinician exploits these paradoxes. Your colleague says, "I took over the care of a nice old chap today. He's got congestive heart failure. But some fool put him on beta-blockers. Just what he doesn't need — depressed myocardial contractility." You reply, "I know exactly what you mean. I used to go around warning patients with CHF to avoid beta-blockers like the plague. Turns out they would have done better to avoid me. Beta-blockers actually reduce mortality in CHF! I think it may be time for us old folks to unlearn a thing or two."

Conclusion

In this paper we presented 8 techniques that may be of help in dealing with a colleague who is, well, um, wrong. If employed properly and used judiciously, these techniques may help avoid embarrassment for all and might even allow you to convey some valuable information. Perhaps one day hospital disciplinary committees might also adopt some of these points of diplomacy. Furthermore, by using these approaches, you may be able to create for yourself a reservoir of good will among your colleagues. This may prove to be of immense help when *you* make a mistake.

Reprinted with permission of the Canadian Medical Association Journal.
This article was originally published in:
CMAJ • DEC. 12, 2000; 163 (12) 1570 — 1572

Chapter 2. Deconstructing Pooh

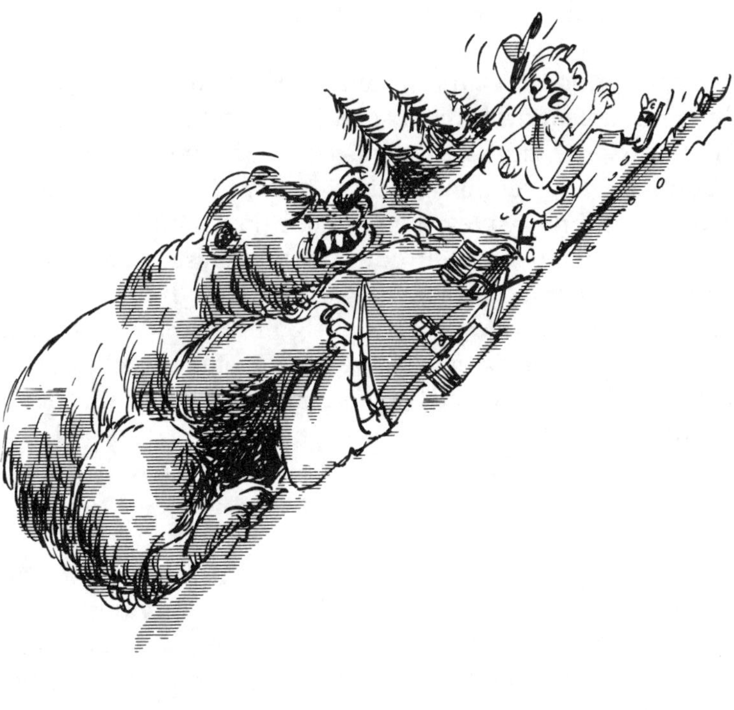

Pathology in the Hundred Acre Wood: a neurodevelopmental perspective on A.A. Milne

Sarah E. Shea, Kevin Gordon, Ann Hawkins,
Janet Kawchuk, and Donna Smith

Somewhere at the top of the hundred acre wood a little boy and his bear play. On the surface it is an innocent world, but on closer examination by our group of experts we find a forest where neurodevelopmental and psychosocial problems go unrecognized and untreated.

On the surface it is an innocent world: Christopher Robin, living in a beautiful forest surrounded by his loyal animal friends. Generations of readers of A.A. Milne's Winnie-the-Pooh stories have enjoyed these seemingly benign tales.[1,2] However, perspectives change with time, and it is clear to our group of modern neurodevelopmentalists that these are in fact stories of Seriously Troubled Individuals, many of whom meet DSM-IV[3] criteria for significant disorders (Table 1). We have done an exhaustive review of the works of A.A. Milne and offer our conclusions about the inhabitants of the Hundred Acre Wood in hopes that our observations will help the medical community understand that there is a Dark Underside to this world.

We begin with Pooh. This unfortunate bear embodies the concept of comorbidity. Most striking is his Attention Deficit Hyperactivity Disorder (ADHD), inattentive subtype. As clinicians, we had some debate about whether Pooh might also demonstrate significant impulsivity, as witnessed, for example, by his poorly thought out attempt to get honey by disguising himself as a rain cloud. We concluded, however, that this reflected more on his comorbid cognitive impairment, further aggravated by an obsessive fixation on honey. The latter, of course, has also contributed to his significant obesity. Pooh's perseveration on food and his repetitive counting behaviours raise the diagnostic possibility of Obsessive Compulsive Disorder (OCD). Given his coexisting ADHD and OCD, we question whether Pooh may over time present with Tourette's syndrome. Pooh is also clearly described as having Very Little Brain. We could not confidently diagnose microcephaly, however, as we do not know whether standards exist for the head circumference of the brown bear. The cause of Pooh's poor brain growth may be found in the stories themselves. Early on we see Pooh being dragged downstairs bump, bump, bump, on the back of his head. Could his later cognitive struggles be the result of a type of Shaken Bear Syndrome?

Pooh needs intervention. We feel drugs are in order. We cannot but wonder how much richer Pooh's life might be were he to have a trial of low-dose stimulant medication. With the right supports, including methylphenidate, Pooh might be fitter and more functional and perhaps produce (and remember) more poems.

I take a
PILL-tiddley pom
It keeps me
STILL-tiddley pom,
It keeps me
STILL-tiddley pom
Not
fiddling.

And what of little Piglet? Poor, anxious, blushing, flustered little Piglet. He clearly suffers from a Generalized Anxiety Disorder. Had he been appropriately assessed and his condition diagnosed when he was young, he might have been placed on an antipanic agent, such as paroxetine, and been saved from the emotional trauma he experienced while attempting to trap heffalumps.

Pooh and Piglet are at risk for additional self-esteem injury because of the chronic dysthymia of their neighbour, Eeyore. What a sad life that donkey lives. We do not have sufficient history to diagnose this as an inherited, endogenous depression or to know whether some early trauma contributed to his chronic negativism, low energy and anhe(haw)donia. Eeyore would benefit greatly from an antidepressant, perhaps combined with individual therapy. Maybe with a little fluoxetine, Eeyore might see the humour
in the whole tail-losing episode. Even if a patch of St. John's wort grew near his thistles, the forest could ring with a braying laugh.

Our neurodevelopmental group agrees about poor Owl: obviously bright, but dyslexic. His poignant attempts to cover up for his phonological deficits are similar to what we see day in and day out in others so afflicted. If only his condition had been identified early and he received more intensive support!

We especially worry about baby Roo. It is not his impulsivity or hyperactivity that concerns us, as we feel that those are probably age appropriate. We worry about the environment in which he is developing. Roo is growing up in a single-parent household, which puts him at high risk for Poorer Outcome. We predict we will someday see a delinquent, jaded, adolescent Roo hanging out late at night at the top of the forest, the ground littered with broken bottles of extract of malt and the butts of smoked thistles. We think that this will be Roo's reality, in part because of a second issue. Roo's closest friend is Tigger, who is *not* a good Role Model. Peer influences strongly affect outcome.

Table 1: DSM-IV multiaxial diagnosis of conditions demonstrated by the inhabitants of the Hundred Acre Wood

Inhabitant	**Axis I** Clinical disorders	**Axis II** Personality disorders/ mental retardation	**Axis III** General medical conditions	**Axis IV** Psychosocial/ environmental problems
Winnie-the-Pooh	ADHD, inattentive subtype; OCD (provisional diagnosis)	Borderline intellectual functioning (Very Little Brain)	Poor diet, obesity, binge eating	-
Piglet	Generalized anxiety disorder	-	Failure to thrive	-
Eeyore	Dysthymic disorder	-	Traumatic amputation of tail	Housing problems
Rabbit	-	Narcissistic personality disorder	-	-
Owl	Reading disorder	-	-	Housing problems
Tigger	ADHD, hyperactivity-impulsivity subtype	-	-	-
Kanga	-	-	-	Single parent, unemployed, overprotective of child
Roo	-	-	-	Single parenthood, undesirable peer group, victim of unusual feeding practices (extract of malt)
Christopher Robin	Gender identity disorder of childhood (provisional diagnosis)	-	-	Lack of parental supervision, possible educational problems

Note: ADHD = attention deficit hyperactivity disorder, OCD = obsessive compulsive disorder.
*The Axis V (global assessment of functioning) scale was deferred.

We acknowledge that Tigger is gregarious and affectionate, but he has a recurrent pattern of risk-taking behaviours. Look, for example, at his impulsive sampling of unknown substances when he first comes to the Hundred Acre Wood. With the mildest of provocation he tries honey, haycorns and even thistles. Tigger has no knowledge of the potential outcome of his experimentation.

Later we find him climbing tall trees and acting in a way that can only be described as socially intrusive. He leads Roo into danger. Our clinical group has had its own debate about what the best medication might be for Tigger. Some of us have argued that his behaviours, occurring in a context of obvious hyperactivity and impulsivity, would suggest the need for a stimulant medication. Others have wondered whether clonidine might be helpful, or perhaps a combination of the two. Unfortunately we could not answer the question as scientifically as we would have liked because we could find only human studies in the literature. Even if we were able to help Tigger, we would still have the problem of Roo's growing up with a single parent. Kanga is noted to be somewhat overprotective. Could her possessiveness of Roo relate to a previous run-in with social services? And where will Kanga be in the future? It is highly likely that she will end up older, blowsier, struggling to look after several joeys conceived in casual relationships with different fathers, stuck at a dead end with inadequate financial resources. But perhaps we are being too gloomy. Kanga may prove to be one of those exceptional single mothers who show a natural resilience — an ability, if we may say so, to bounce back. Maybe Kanga will pass her high school equivalency test, earn a university degree and maybe even get an MBA. Perhaps some day Kanga will buy the Hundred Acre Wood and develop it into a gated community of $500,000 homes. But that is not likely to happen, particularly in a social context that does not appear to value education and provides no strong female leadership. What leadership there is in the Hundred Acre Wood is simply that offered by one small boy, Christopher Robin. Our group believes that Christopher Robin has not exhibited any diagnosable condition as yet, but we are concerned about several issues. There is the obvious problem of a complete absence of parental supervision, not to mention the fact that this child is spending his time talking to animals. We also noted in the stories early signs of difficulty with academics and felt that E.H. Shepard's illustrations suggest possible future gender identity issues for this child. The more psychoanalytical member in our group indicated that there could be some Freudian meaning to his peculiar naming of his bear as Winnie-the-Pooh.

Finally, we turn to Rabbit. We note his tendency to be extraordinarily self-important and his odd belief system that he has a great many relations (many of other species!) and friends. He seems to have an overriding need to organize others, often against their will, into new groupings, alwayswith himself at the top of the reporting structure. We believe that he has missed his calling, as he clearly belongs in senior-level hospital administration. Somewhere at the top of the forest a little boy and his bear play. Sadly, the forest is not, in fact, a place of enchantment, but rather one of disenchantment, where neurodevelopmental and psychosocial problems go unrecognized and untreated. It is unfortunate that an Expotition was never Organdized to a Child Development Clinic.

References

1. Milne AA. *Winnie-the-Pooh*. London: Methuen; 1926.
2. Milne AA. *The House at Pooh Corner*. London: Methuen; 1928.
3. American Psychiatric Association. *Diagnostic and statistical manual of mental disorders.* 4th ed. Washington: APA; 1994.

Reprinted with permission of the Canadian Medical Association Journal.
This article was originally published in:
CMAJ • DEC. 12, 2000; 163 (12) 1557 — 1559

From the files of Dr. Grinch:

A Psychiatric Interpretation of 'Twas the Night Before Christmas

David J. Robinson, M.D.

'Twas the night before Christmas, when all through the house, Not a creature has stirring, not even a mouse.

Consider a drug-induced catatonic stupor involving the whole family. Could this be delusional rodent infestation?

The stockings were hung by the chimney with care,
In hopes that St. Nicholas soon would be there;

This may be a dominant figure (cult leader?) demanding certain rituals be fulfilled before his return — he seems to make an unusual request for warm leggings.

The children were nestled, all snug in their beds,
While visions of sugar plums danced in their heads;

Visual hallucinations. Check to see if the kid's hot chocolate was laced with LSD.

And Mama in her 'kerchief and I in my cap,
Had just settled down for long winter's nap,

Doesn't this guy work during the winter? Get income tax and welfare records.

When out on the lawn there arose such a clatter,
I sprang from the bed to see what was the matter.

Check wife for sleep apnea. Is he experiencing auditory hallucinations?

Away to the window I flew like a flash,
Tore open the shutters and threw up the sash.

New-onset sociopathic tendencies; may also be hyperactive. He's got to switch to decaf and reduce intake after dinner.

The moon on the breast of the new-fallen snow,
Gave a luster of mid-day to objects below.

Visual illusions in addition to the auditory hallucinations. This fellow requires a complete medical investigation — fire up the CT scanner!

When what to my wondering eyes should appear,
But a miniature sleigh and eight tiny reindeer.

He's definitely lost it. Lilliputian hallucinations are a particularly bad sign. What is it with these animal images? First mice, now reindeer. . . hope this isn't Equus.

With a little old driver so lively and quick,
I knew in a moment it must be St. Nick.

Is this a drug dealer? The cult leader? He seems manic.

More rapid than eagles his coursers they came,
And he whistled, and shouted, and called them by name:

Bingo. Anyone flying around a strange area whistling and shouting at this time of night must have a mood disorder.

"Now, Dasher! now, Dancer! now, Prancer and Vixen!
On Comet! on, Cupid! on, Donder and Blitzen!

Where is Rudolph? Something is wrong here.

To the top of the porch! To the top of the wall!
Now dash away! dash away! dash away all!"

That was quick. . . impulse control appears to be poor. Possible intermittent explosive disorder.

As dry leaves that before the wild hurricane fly,
When they meet with an obstacle, mount to the sky,

Just what are those "dry leaves?" Where's his stash?

So up to the house-top the coursers they flew,
With a sleigh full of toys, and St. Nicholas too.

This man is highly disorganized and regressed. At least he brought his own toys.

And then, in a twinkling, I heard on the roof
The prancing and pawing of each little hoof.

Back to those auditory hallucinations. . . where are the results of his scan?

As I drew in my head and was turning around,
Down the chimney St. Nicholas came with a bound.

Unusual method of entry. . . uses the element of surprise on unsuspecting victims. He must really want those warm socks.

He was dressed all in fur from his head to his foot,
And his clothes were all tarnished with ashes and soot;

Is he unkempt? Disheveled? Any other negative signs?

A bundle of toys he had flung on his back,
And he looked like a peddler just opening his pack,

> And just what is in that pack?

His eyes — how they twinkled! His dimples how merry!
His cheeks were like roses, his nose like a cherry!

> Perhaps his brain got frostbite along the way too.

His droll little mouth was drawn like a bow,
And the beard on his chin was as white as the snow;

> He seems to disarm others with his aged appearance.

The stump of a pipe he held tight in his teeth,
And the smoke, it encircled his head like a wreath;

> After projecting this grandfatherly visage, he poisons the air supply, causing a drug-induced state of compliance.

He had a broad face and a round little belly,
That shook when he laughed, like a bowl full of jelly.

> Truncal obesity. . . round face. . . sounds a little Cushingoid.

He was chubby and plump, a right jolly old elf,
And I laughed when I saw him, in spite of myself.

> Oh yeah, well watch out for the food left on the counter!

A wink of an eye and a twist of his head,
Soon gave me to know I had nothing to dread.

> There appears to be some delusional misinterpretation of these body movements.

He spoke not a word, but went straight to his work,
And filled all the stockings; then turned with a jerk,

His fix must be wearing off — he's getting irritable.

And laying a finger aside of his nose,
And giving a nod, up the chimney he rose.

More secret signals. . . this may be post-hypnotic suggestion rendering automatic obedience from his followers.

He sprang to his sleigh, to his team gave a whistle,
And away they all flew like the down of a thistle.

A brief appearance helps keep up the mystique. If they ask too many questions, he'll blow his cover.

But I heard him exclaim, ere he drove out of sight,
"Happy Christmas to all, and to all a good-night!"

And so the cycle continues . . .

Assessment

This household appears to be part of a large following (possibly a cult) performing an elaborate ritual in the hope of receiving an important visit. After putting his children to bed and attempting to sleep himself, the narrator/victim is deluged by abnormal perceptions. While stumbling around chasing his hallucinations, the narrator/victim is confronted by the cult leader, who uses surprise tactics and post-hypnotic suggestion to assuage alarm. While control of the followers may be partly pharmacologically-induced, the cult leader may well have a diagnosable mood disorder or a serious medical problem. This charismatic central figure appears to use behavioral methods (intermittent rewards) as a means of securing the allegiance of his followers.

Because Politically Correct Isn't the Only "P.C."

Psychiatrically Correct Comics

David J. Robinson, M.D.

Calvin and Hobbes	Calvinist and his Imaginary Companion
Spiderman	Arachnomania
Superman	The Intergalactic Narcissist
Beetle Bailey	The Military Chronicles of a Self-Defeating Personality
Peanuts	The Childhood Histories of an Avoidant Personality, his Borderline Girlfriend, a Schizoid Pianist, and a Socially-Disinhibited Canine
Dennis the Menace	Misadventures of the Neighborhood's Conduct-Disordered Boy
The Far Side	Posttraumatic Zoophilia
Doonesbury	Intellectualization Illustrated
Cathy	The Ranting of a Diet-Obsessed, Dysthymic, Dependent Personality
Dilbert	The Inadequate Personality in the Workplace
Herman	The Journal of Concrete Thinking

The Simpsons	The Familial Consequences of the Brainstem being the Highest Cortical Center for Decision Making
Beavis & Butthead	Two Inner Children that Escaped from Inner Day Care
Outland	Adventures in Primary Process
Hagar	Conquests of an Antisocial Viking
Garfield	Trials of a Passive-Aggressive Feline

TV's Original Dysfunctional Family Unit:

The Brady Bunch as the Template for Family Disaster

David J. Robinson, M.D.

The Brady Bunch was a sitcom that aired between 1969 and 1974. This supposedly "family-oriented" show featured one-hundred-and-seventeen episodes of thirty minutes duration that took up a prime time spot on Friday nights for the duration of its run. The premise of the show was the integration of two broken family units: a man with three sons and a woman with three daughters. The show was very popular during its initial airing and continues to be a favorite among re-runs. On the surface, this show, which was targeted at children, appeared to deal with rather banal issues (such as slumber parties, tattling on one another, celebrity worship, sibling rivalry etc.).

In reality, this show was a catalyst for causing the widespread dysfunction in families in the decades that followed. Through its unassuming "groovy" appeal and use of subliminal persuasion, this show went on to wreak havoc in the lives of generations of its viewers.

Since this show was created, the divorce rate has sky-rocketed. Viewers of the series were influenced into thinking that the Brady Bunch was the way families *should* be composed. First marriages soon became like warm-up tosses in horseshoes; they just didn't count. The generation exposed to this show became single-mindedly intent on finding a spouse, having six children, dividing them up along gender lines, and then separating. The family planning consequences of this goal have led to overpopulation and wide-spread esteem problems in cases where the proper number of boys or girls didn't come along. The Brady Bunch even spawned a more outrageous spin-off called, "Eight is Enough."

Despite the sugar-coated approach to family life portrayed in the Brady Bunch, there were key issues that were simply not discussed, such as parental loss or the nurturing requirements of six needy children. Despite these glaring omissions in programming, there were deficiencies in the storyline that unequivocally reveal this show as the template for family dysfunction.

- **The fate of Carol Brady's first husband was never revealed.**

Clearly this loss was traumatic enough without it being shrouded in mystery. Mrs. Brady never took the time to inform her new family about the loss of her daughters' father. The absence of revealing this man's fate speaks volumes about Carol Brady. Rather than being involved in bereavement counseling with her daughters, she indulges her histrionic personality style by repressing his exit from her life. This also raises the possibility that she was an axe murderer and needed to conceal this man's fate in order to attract another husband/victim.

- **The city the Brady's lived in was never mentioned.**

This was a ratings-motivated attempt to appeal to all viewers. The Brady's were fashioned to be "any family" from "any city" in the USA. Denying such basic identifying features as the place of residence for the sake of popularity further reveals the pathology of this family. Trying to convince everyone to like you by not saying anything about yourself sets a deplorable example. It only influences viewers to suffer from the same inane, acceptance-focused drive that affected these people. This carefully scripted omission perpetuates the stereotype of "image over substance" that plagues the post-Brady era.

• When Mike Brady designed the house, why didn't he include more bedrooms for the children?

Mike was purportedly an architect, not a high school drafting drop-out. In this house of eight people, he included only three bedrooms. One for Carol and himself (naturally), one for all three girls and another for the three boys. Did either of these parents understand the inherent dangers in having both latency stage and genital stage children in the same room? Of course not! They were too busy trying to preach a brand of "Aesops's Fables" morality to their children after the fact. By allowing this kind of rooming situation to occur, the Brady's unconsciously encouraged their children to act out in order to have a theme for each episode. Inducing their children to misbehave and then punishing them for it set up a double bind that kept the children from asking for more humane living arrangements. Instead of engaging in preventative measures that would foster the development of each child as an individual, these parents stunted the emotional growth of their children in order to gratify their own needs.

• The fate of the Brady's pets was never revealed.

A large number of animals appeared on the Brady Bunch. The pets most prominently featured were Tiger the dog and Fluffy the cat. Too immersed in their own image as the perfect family, it only took the Brady's until the third show to start vilifying their pets. Poor Tiger is blamed for one of the children's obvious kleptomania as both a doll and a kazoo go missing in a single episode.

Things go so poorly for the Brady animals that when Tiger

fathers a litter of puppies, he cannot bear to have them born at home. As early as the first season, the pets were being "deleted" from the script. Their fate is still unknown.

It is interesting to note that movie producers include a statement in the credits that no animals were harmed during filming and that there were people looking out for the animals' welfare. No such notice is given at the end of Brady Bunch episodes.

• What precisely happened when Greg kept a goat overnight in his room?

In later years, the Brady parents had done so much moralizing that they themselves were sick of hearing their lessons. How far did things deteriorate? Well, in the final season, Greg (the oldest boy) stole Raquel the goat, the mascot of a rival football team. The Bradys must have had some idea about Greg's twisted fetishes because at this point in the series they had given him a private room in the attic. Where the Brady Bunch could have launched a groundbreaking episode dealing with the recognition and acceptance of Greg's bestiality, the evening in question was merely swept under the rug, as were so many issues in the Brady household.

Other areas of concern for future discussion are as follows:

- Great Grandmother Brady was arrested for indecent exposure
- What is the focus on this "hair of gold" for? This focus Aryan tendencies demands fuller a examination
- Why didn't we ever get to see Mike and Carol's bathroom?
- Did Alice ever get a day off? What kind of duress was she placed under to constantly ignore her own needs?
- Bananas come in bunches, families don't. Who's idea was this anyway?

Chapter 3. Diagnostic Shortcuts

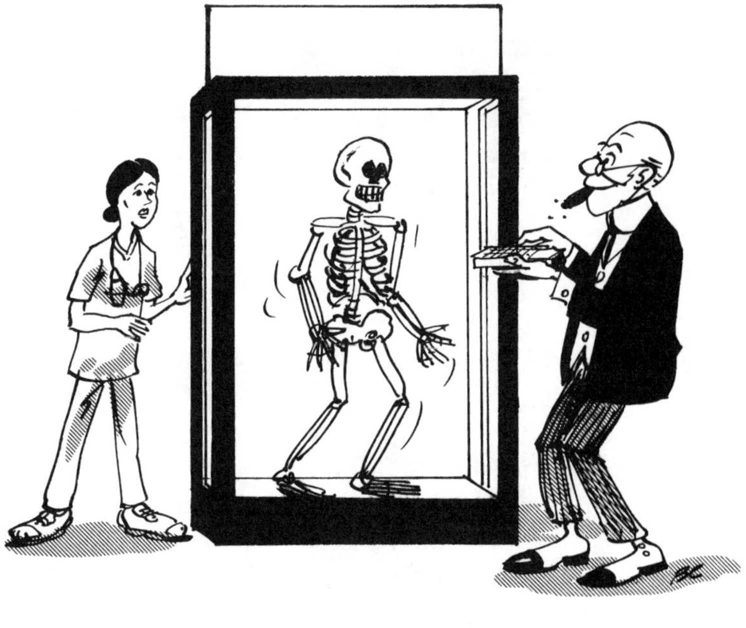

Initial Diagnosis I

David J. Robinson, M.D. & Donna L. Robinson, M.D.

A common practice in case presentations is to disguise the identifying features of patients. One of the most practical methods of doing this has been to use the person's initials. The authors propose that choosing initials related to the diagnosis not only preserves confidentiality, but also thwarts those sadistic enough to conceal essential information until the end of the presentation.

Initials	Diagnosis
T.V.	Paraphilia
K.Y.	Paraphilia
I.F.	Obsessive-Compulsive Disorder
Z.Z.	Narcolepsy
B.S.	Confabulating
I.D.	Fugue State
M.I.	Hypochondriasis
H.I.	Mania
U.P.	Mania
O.K.	Euthymic Mood State
L.O.	Depression
R.X.	Prescription Medication Abuse
R.I.	Lilliputian Delusions
I.V.	Substance Abuser
E.X.	Adjustment Disorder
A.X.	Intermittent Explosive Disorder
T.B.	Somatization Disorder
A.D.	Math Phobia
L.B.	Anorexia Nervosa
L.L.	Friend or enemy of Superman

Initial Diagnosis II

David J. Robinson, M.D. & Donna L. Robinson, M.D.

Initials	Diagnosis
X.X.	Antisocial Personality
I.d.	Antisocial Personality
E.Z.	Avoidant Personality
N.O.	Avoidant Personality
F.U.	Borderline Personality
F.O.	Borderline Personality
O.D.	Borderline Personality
I.Q.	Obsessive-Compulsive Personality
I.E.	Obsessive-Compulsive Personality
C.O.	Dependent Personality
C.U.	Dependent Personality
X.O.	Histrionic Personality
B.B.	Histrionic Personality
M.E.	Narcissistic Personality
N.B.	Narcissistic Personality
I.M.	Narcissistic Personality
X.S.	Narcissistic Personality
M.Y.	Narcissistic Personality
X.L.	Narcissistic Personality
D.A.	Paranoid Personality
Q.T.	Paranoid Personality
M.O.	Paranoid Personality
S.O.	Passive-Aggressive Personality
O.T.	Passive-Aggressive Personality
G.O.	Schizoid Personality
I.T.	Schizoid Personality
E.T.	Schizotypal Personality
O.Z.	Schizotypal Personality
B.O.	Unkempt Character
P.U.	Disheveled Character

Psychler Pathology

David J. Robinson, M.D.

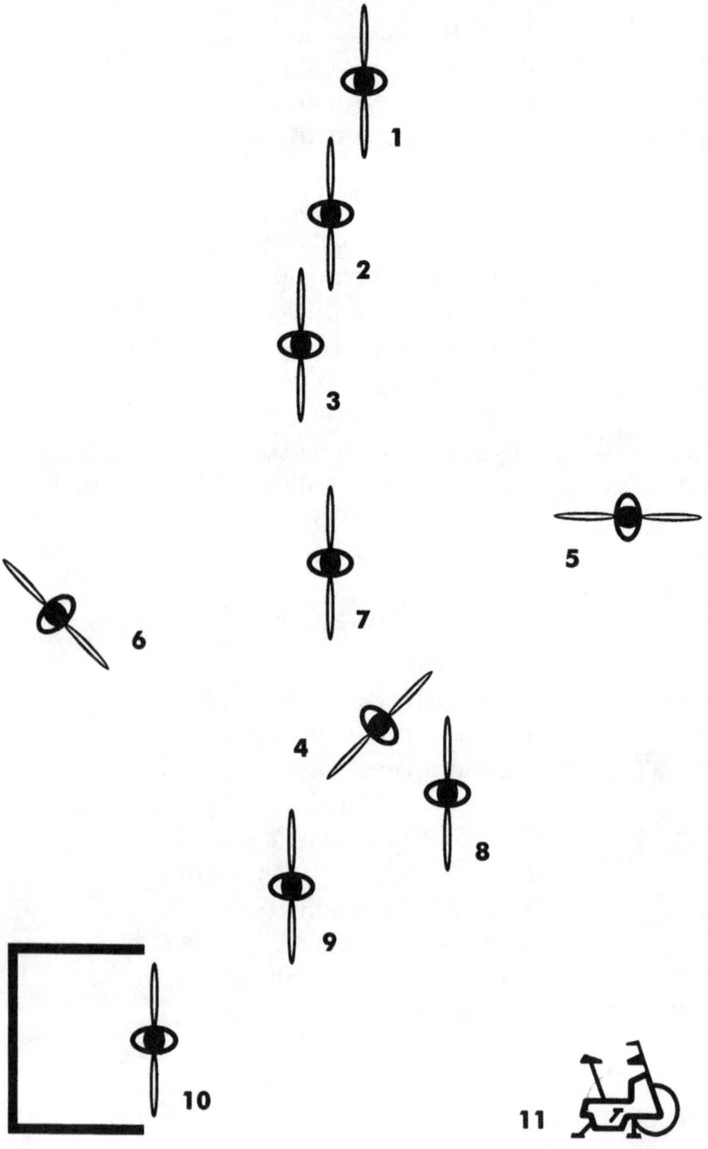

Key

1. **Identity:** Narcissistic Personality
Rides: Custom-built titanium frame racer
Activity: Leader of pack, even if only for the first mile

2. **Identity:** Histrionic Personality
Rides: Trés chic model with neon decals and streamers
Activity: Stays close to her man (currently sharing a mirror with the Narcissist); being in front also gets the attention of the other riders

3. **Identity:** Borderline Personality
Rides: Hybrid (due to identity diffusion)
Activity: Slashes tires of Histrionic ahead of her

4. **Identity:** Passive-Aggressive Personality
Rides: BMX with pedals modified to stop others from passing
Activity: Drafts others for whole race, then cuts them off at the end

5. **Identity:** Antisocial Personality
Rides: Grunge Mountain Bike with studded tires
Activity: Departs from race so stolen bike doesn't get noticed

6. **Identity:** Schizotypal Personality
Rides: Recumbent
Activity: Heads off beaten path; looks for trinkets along road

7. **Identity:** Dependent Personality
Rides: Mo-ped (to be able to maintain any speed)
Activity: Stays in the center of the pack — always

8. **Identity:** Avoidant Personality
Rides: Modified Tricycle
Activity: Lets others get ahead so they invite him back

9. **Identity:** Paranoid Personality
Rides: Armored three speed
Activity: Stays behind to keep an eye on everyone else

10. **Identity:** Obsessive-Compulsive Personality
Rides: Techno-weenie Special with 500 page manual
Activity: Must get tire pressure perfect before using bike

11. **Identity:** Schizoid Personality
Rides: Stationary Cycle
Activity: Sees *le monde à la maision*

Birth Trauma Revisited:

A Theory of Psychiatric Presentation

Lewis H. Richmond, M.D.
San Antonio, Texas

The author, through extensive personal research, proposes that the type of presentation of an infant at birth influences subsequent psychological development. The following forms of presentation are of particular significance, and listed with their corresponding psychiatric condition or symptom.

Presentation	Diagnosis
Wrinkled brow (may include furrowed brow)	Depression
Tongue	Paraphilia
Nose	Olfactory Hallucinations
Ear	Auditory Hallucinations
Breech (buttocks)	Passive-Aggressive Personality Disorder
Eye	Paranoid Personality Disorder
Umbilical cord	Dependent Personality Disorder
Foot in mouth	Inadequate Personality Disorder
Crawls back in	Agoraphobia

Fist	Intermittent Explosive Disorder
Variety of lies	Antisocial Personality Disorder
Staring at reflection in amniotic fluid	Narcissistic Personality Disorder
No presentation	Schizoid Personality Disorder
Several parts presenting simultaneously	Multiple Personality Disorder
Hands over head	Avoidant Personality Disorder
Cigar	Neo-Freudian

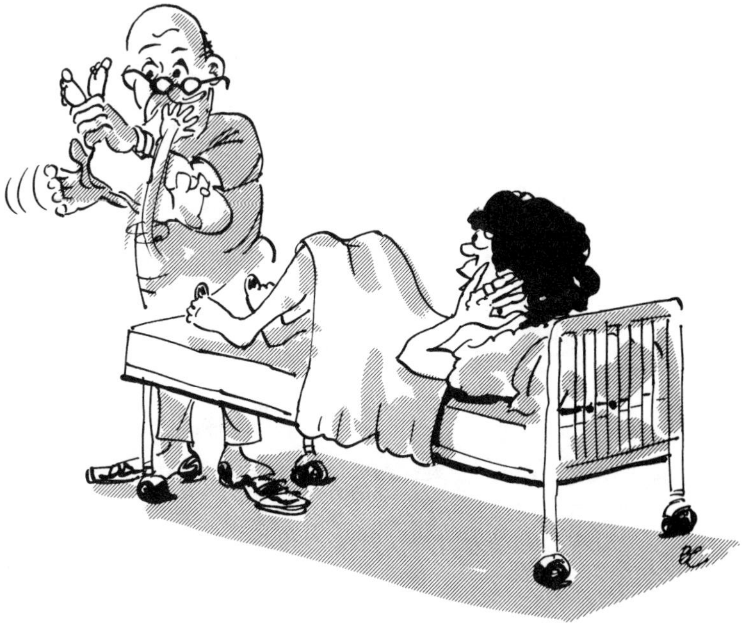

DSM Bumper Stickers

Rohan Robertson, M.D. & Josie Pressacco, M.D.

- You're never down and out with Delusions of Grandeur.
- With Alzheimer's, you make new friends every day.
- You're never redundant with obsessive-compulsive disorder.
- You're never redundant with obsessive-compulsive disorder.
- Don't be minimized by Anorexia Nervosa.
- With Bulimia, you can stomach anything.
- You're always running scared with Phobic Disorder.
- There's always a full house with Multiple Personality Disorder.
- You're never a real pain with Somatoform Disorder.
- If you've got Kleptomania, then take something for it.
- Wanna bet you can quit gambling?
- If you're paranoid, lead the way!
- If you're an Obsessive-Compulsive Personality, work it out!
- Panic attacks are a cause for alarm!

The Wheel of Misfortune:

The Adolescent-O-Meter

Michael F. Shaughnessy, Ph.D. & Teresa Naggs
Portales, New Mexico

Parents and guardians are often concerned about what is bothering their teenagers. Adolescents however, are often loath to even acknowledge their parents, much less talk about what's going on. In order to rectify this situation, the authors, one a practicing psychologist, and the second, a practicing parent, have developed the **Adolescent-O-Meter**. This device allows teenagers to simply move the arrow on a wheel, pointing to whatever is bothering them on a specific day. This device can be attached to a teenager's door and readjusted on a daily or even hourly basis. The meter also has a blank space if the reason that they are cranky, bellicose, stuporous, bush-whacked or psychotic on a specific day isn't specified. Since the causative factors in adolescent difficulties are generally viewed as beyond adult comprehension, up to three levels of complexity are provided in this example.

Initial Complaint:

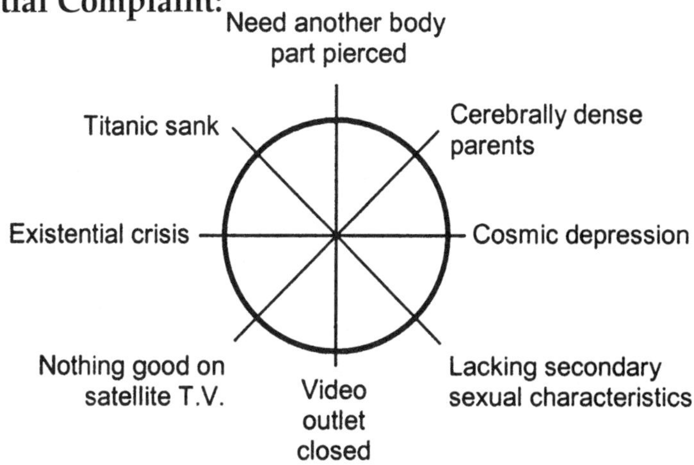

Due To:

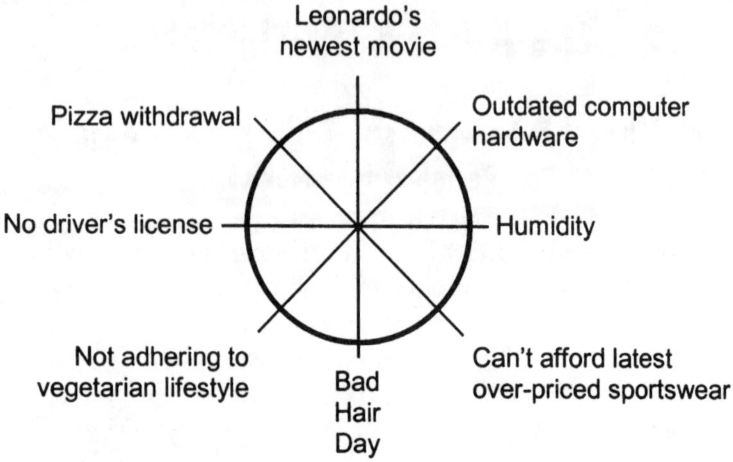
Leonardo's newest movie
Outdated computer hardware
Humidity
Can't afford latest over-priced sportswear
Bad Hair Day
Not adhering to vegetarian lifestyle
No driver's license
Pizza withdrawal

Due To:

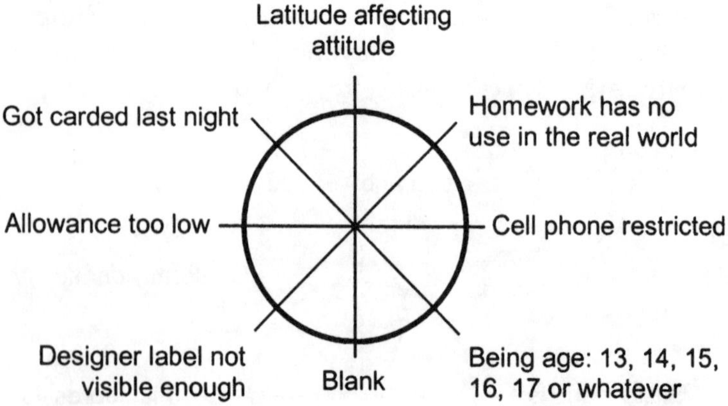
Latitude affecting attitude
Homework has no use in the real world
Cell phone restricted
Being age: 13, 14, 15, 16, 17 or whatever
Blank
Designer label not visible enough
Allowance too low
Got carded last night

Chapter 4. Light Bulb Jokes

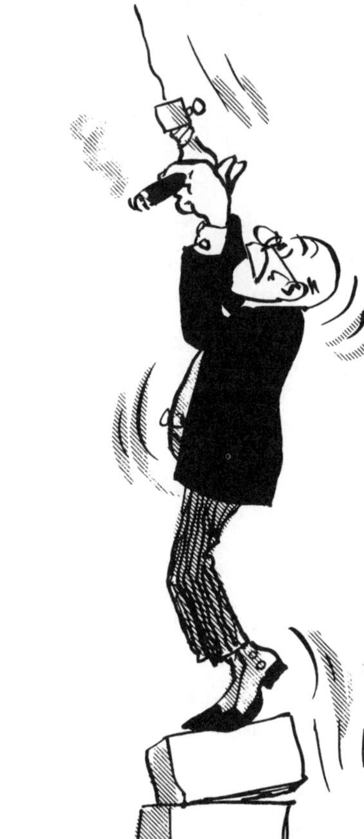

Psychiatrists

How many psychiatrists does it take to change a light bulb?
- None. Psychiatrists aren't afraid of the dark.
- None. The light bulb will change when it's ready.
- None. Psychiatrists don't change light bulbs.
- None. There never actually was a light bulb.

- One. But the light bulb really has to want to change.
- Just one, but it takes nine visits.

- Two. One to screw it almost all the way in and another to give it a surprise twist at the end.
- Two. One to change the bulb and the other to tell her that she's changing it the wrong way

- Three. One to find a bulb specialist, one to find a bulb installation specialist, and one to bill it all to Medicare.

How many psychoanalysts does it take to change a light bulb?
- Why does the light bulb necessarily have to change?
- How many do you think it takes?
- It depends on what you want to change it into.
- What kind of answer did you have in mind?
- How many can you afford?

How many Freudians does it take to change a light bulb?
- Two. One to change the bulb and one to hold the penis. . . I mean ladder!

Psychology Internet Mail List Subscribers

How many psychologist internet mail list subscribers does it take to change a light bulb?
- 1 to change the light bulb and to post to the mail list that the light bulb has been changed
- 14 to share similar experiences of changing light bulbs and how the light bulb could have been changed differently
- 7 to caution about the dangers of changing light bulbs

- 28 to point out spelling/grammar errors in posts about changing light bulbs.
- 53 to flame the spell checkers
- 156 to write to the list administrator complaining about the light bulb discussion and its inappropriateness to this mail list
- 41 to correct spelling in the spelling/grammar flames
- 109 to post that this list is not about light bulbs and to please take this email exchange to alt.lite.bulb
- 203 to demand that cross posting to alt.grammar, alt.spelling and alt.punctuation about changing light bulbs be stopped
- 111 to defend the posting to this list saying that we all use light bulbs and therefore the posts *are* relevant to this mail list
- 306 to debate which method of changing light bulbs is superior, where to buy the best light bulbs, what brand of light bulbs work best for this technique, and what brands are faulty
- 27 to post URLs where one can see examples of different light bulbs
- 14 to post that the URLs were posted incorrectly, and to post corrected URLs
- 3 to post about links they found from the URLs that are relevant to this list which makes light bulbs relevant to this list
- 33 to concatenate all posts to date, then quote them including all headers and footers, and then add "Me Too."
- 12 to post to the list that they are unsubscribing because they cannot handle the light bulb controversy
- 19 to quote the "Me Too's" to say, "Me Three"
- 4 to suggest that posters request the light bulb FAQ
- 1 to propose new alt.change.lite.bulb newsgroup
- 47 to say this is just what alt.physic.cold_fusion was meant for, leave it here
- 143 votes for alt.lite.bulb

(author unknown)

Personality Disorders

How many schizotypal personalities does it take to change a light bulb?

- None. Schizotypals carry their own light.
- To get to the other side.

How many schizoid personalities does it take to change a light bulb?

- All of them.
- None. There is nothing to change.

How many paranoid personalities does it take to change a light bulb?

- None. The light bulb contains the seeds of its own revolution.
- Fifty. One to screw in the light bulb and 49 to guard him.

How many antisocial personalities does it take to change a light bulb?

- None. They never see the light anyway.
- Three. One to change the bulb, one to be a witness, and one to shoot the witness.

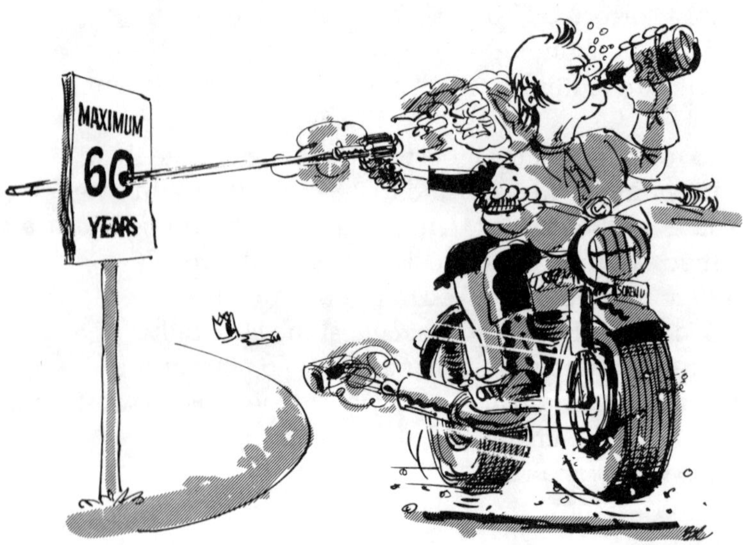

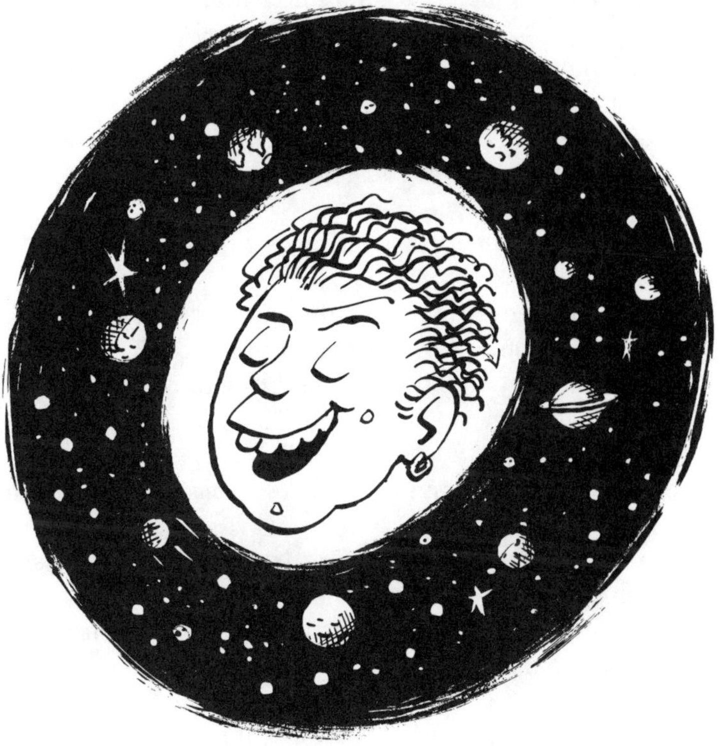

How many narcissistic personalities does it take to change a light bulb?

- One and only one. They don't like to share the spotlight.
- Just one. He grabs the bulb and waits for the world to revolve around him.

How many borderline personalities does it take to change a light bulb?

- Only one, but it takes a lot of light bulbs!
- Five. One to change the bulb and four to pull the ladder out from under her.

How many histrionic personalities does it take to change a light bulb?

- Two. One to mix a drink and the other to arrange for a contractor.
- Twenty. One to change the bulb, two to turn the ladder, and seventeen on the guest list.

How many avoidant personalities does it take to change a light bulb?

- None. They never change light bulbs in case someone enters the room who wants to sit in the dark.
- Two. One to change the bulb and one to not change the bulb.

How many dependent personalities does it take to change a light bulb?

• Two. One to change the bulb, and one to write a song about how good the old light bulb was.

• Six. One to turn the bulb, one for support, and four to relate to the experience.

How many obsessive-compulsive personalities does it take to change a light bulb?

- None. Technically speaking, obsessive-compulsive personalities only replace dark bulbs.
- Just one. But he has to check it 100 times, once for each watt.
- Two. One to screw in the bulb and one to fend off all the dependent personalities trying to share the experience
- Fewer than it takes to change a heavy bulb.

How many passive-aggressive personalities does it take to screw in a light bulb?

- Two. One to assure that everything possible is being done while the other one screws the bulb into the water faucet.
- Two. One to change it and the other to act as a chaperone.

Chapter 5. Managed Relationships

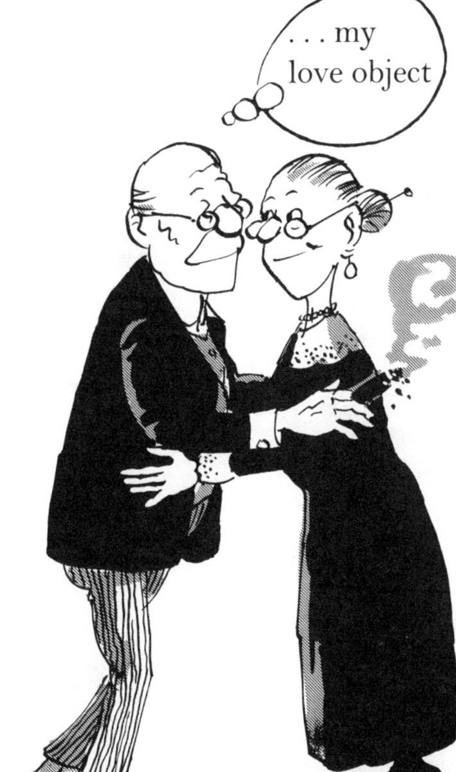

The Theory of S.P.U.R.I.O.U.S. Intelligence

Steven J. Kirsh, Ph.D.
Washburn University

Recently, several theories have been put forth to explain the complex and multifaceted nature of human intelligence. For instance, Robert Sternberg posits three distinct categories of intelligence and Howard Gardner proposes seven types of intelligence. However, the theory of S.P.U.R.I.O.U.S. intelligence is inherently better, because it has eight subtypes of intelligence:

Spousal
Political
Uvula
Remote Control
Intra-Bodily Function
Other-Bodily Function
Unique
Scholastic

Thus, the S.P.U.R.I.O.U.S. Intelligence theory is over twice as good as Sternberg's theory and at least 10% better than Gardner's theory. Similar to Gardner's application of his theory to K-12 education, potential applications of the S.P.U.R.I.O.U.S. intelligence theory are listed here.

Spousal Intelligence

Spousal Intelligence (SI) is the ability to manipulate your significant other without his or her knowledge. Clearly, gender differences are prominent, with women being of superior intelligence and men having borderline retardation. Research shows that female SI increases over the life span of a marriage, whereas male SI decreases precipitously. These gender differences are believed to be genetic. Intervention programs should be avoided at any cost. If men ever figured out what was really going on in their relationships, the divorce rate would sky rocket.

Political Intelligence

Political Intelligence is the ability to get others to lie, cheat and steal in order that you get what you want (or at least get them to say they did it after the deed is discovered. Many presidents were deemed to be geniuses in this area. In addition, as my wonderfully insightful, esteemed Department Chair told me, "kissing up" is considered to be a valued form of PI. Political Intelligence should be taught in the schools at an early age. Not only would teachers enjoy their classes more fully, but the potential financial benefits to these children as adults would be astronomical. In today's society, by the time most adults tap their innate PI abilities, they have passed up on many potential years of promotions and salary increases.

Uvula Intelligence

Uvula intelligence (UI) is knowing what that little thing that hangs down in the back of your throat is called. Bulimics are considered to be of high UI. Geniuses actually know the function of the uvula (this is extremely rare). Though there are no applications of this type of intelligence, it does have high criterion validity. UI has been related ($r > .70$) to the WAIS, SAT, and the Beck Depression Inventory.

Remote Control Intelligence

Remote Control Intelligence (RCI) is the ability to watch two or more shows at the same time. Men seem to be of higher RCI than women. However, gender differences may be accounted for by the fact that married women rarely get a chance to exercise their RCI. Research has indicated that husbands tend to hang on to the remote control as if it were a second phallus. As with Spousal Intelligence, in order to keep millions of marriages intact, most intervention programs are best avoided.

Intra-Bodily Function Intelligence

Intra-Bodily Function Intelligence (IBFI) is that ability to recognize when one has to urinate, and can judge how long they can hold it. Truck drivers are of high IBFI. Low IBFI is indicated if you can't make it through a movie without having to go to the bathroom or are frequently spotted relieving yourself at the side of the interstate. IBFI is believed to decline with age. Although low IBFI has its disadvantages in many situations, it can be a great resource for long staff meetings. The spontaneous facial contractions and leg movements associated with low IBFI have been shown to easily excuse individuals from meetings. The Provorse Point of Discomfort of Bladder Distension (PPDBD) scale is used to measure this intelligence (available upon request).

Extensive research has demonstrated that intervention programs are usually ineffective those with very low IBFI, and sufferers are encouraged to find something on which they can "depend."

Other-Bodily Function Intelligence

Other-Bodily Function Intelligence (OBFI) is the ability to tell when someone else has to go to the bathroom. Preschool teachers and daycare providers are geniuses in this area. Nursing home caretakers, however, tend to be of low intelligence. This intelligence is highly correlated with physical empathy — the ability to feel another's pain.

Unique Intelligence

Unique Intelligence (UI) is that intelligence which is unique to each individual and unmeasurable. This intelligence guarantees that we all are geniuses in our own way. Many members of various departments of education are of high UI. Clearly, the education system needs to continue in the direction that it is going in order to give UI the credit that it is due.

Scholastic Intelligence

Scholastic Intelligence (SI) is the ability to do well in school in subjects like Math and English. This form of intelligence is believed to be of little value to today's society. Recent research suggests that SI appears to be on the decline in the United States. On the other hand, as educators have been suggesting for years, UI appears to be on the rise. In order to keep pace with this trend, college admissions examinations, such as the ACT and SAT, need to bolster scores by at least 25% in order to account for UI.

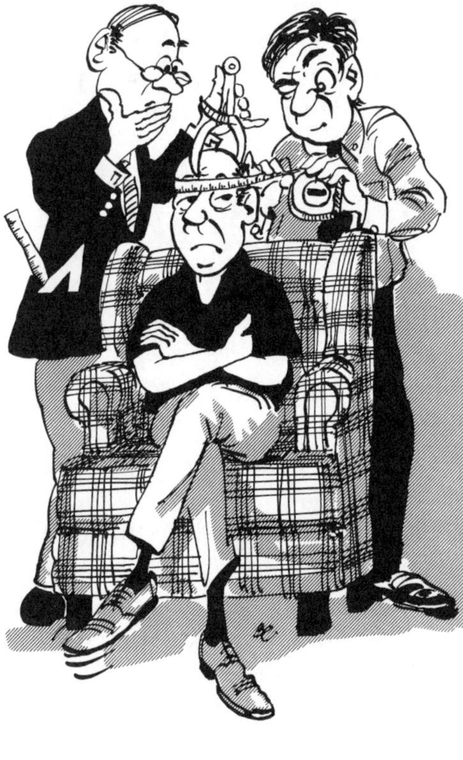

Married Male Memory Loss Syndrome

Steven J. Kirsh, Ph.D.
Geneseo, New York

For centuries, wives have known that their husbands have had problems remembering spousal queries, advice, and admonitions. For instance, recent evidence from the "Dead Sea Scrolls" suggests that in the Garden of Eden, Eve actually told Adam, "I said don't eat the apple. . . you never listen to me." (Anders & Reynolds, 1993). However, it is only recently that psychologists have paid attention to this serious disorder.

It has been estimated that nearly 90% of married men suffer from Married Male Memory Loss Syndrome MMMLS, (Reynolds & Fisher, 1959). What makes this syndrome such a tragedy is that married men do no usually know that they suffer from this disorder until a divorce has been finalized (Trump & Trump, 1990).

MMMLS will be a new clinical disorder listed in the next edition of the Diagnostic and Statistical Manual of Mental Disorders (DSM). The symptoms include:

- Onset immediately after saying "I do"
- Marital Minutiae Amnesia
- Spousal Command Amnesia
- Sports Hypermnesia
- Referral by Spouse for Hearing Check

This paper is being published prior to the release of the next version of the DSM in an attempt to promote the accurate diagnosis of MMMLS so that an effective treatment can be developed. As of yet, there is no known cure for this disorder (Johnson & Griffith, 1977 & 1995).

Clinical Symptoms of MMMLS

In order to be able to diagnose MMMLS, 3 of the 5 symptoms listed above need to be present for a period of at least 6 months.

Onset During Wedding Ceremony

In one of the first studies conducted, Lovett & Roberts (1995), demonstrated that the onset of MMMLS usually occurs during the ceremony itself. In fact, computer analysis of 1000 video tapes indicated that as soon as the groom said, I do, swooning, a loss of balance, or a buckling of the knees typically occurs, which suggests a biological component to MMMLS. Not surprisingly, many men cannot remember taking their vows. In severe cases, the groom, finding himself at the reception, may get drunk, forget he's married, and hit on the maid-of-honor (Arnold & Barr, 1994).

Marital Minutiae Amnesia

One of the hallmark features of MMMLS is the inability to remember details considered to be important to a marriage (Wyman & Reagan, 1949). MMMLS sufferers almost universally cannot remember their anniversary, engagement date, or the first time they made love to their wives. Of note, wives of MMMLS sufferers have developed a coping strategy of engraving important dates on the inside of their husband's wedding bands. Unfortunately, this technique seldom works, for the MMMLS victim either forgets to look or loses the ring.

Importantly, Presley & Presley (1973) identified a warning sign for marital minutia amnesia. They found that prior to the wedding, future victims of MMMLS had difficulty remembering facts associated with the event, e.g., the wedding date and location. Post hoc analyses revealed that most of the brides felt that their grooms' memory loss was the result of "cold feet," which was hoped to disappear after "married bliss."

Spousal Command Amnesia

Almost universally present in this insidious disorder is memory loss for spousal directives. Fortensky & Taylor (1996) found that the most commonly forgotten commands include: taking out the trash, cleaning the dishes, doing the laundry, and putting on a fresh pair of underwear.

Sports "Hypermnesia"

Monroe & DiMaggio (1954) were the first to identify this familiar marker of MMMLS. Their investigation of 792 men revealed that although married men had Marital Minutia Amnesia, their memory for seemingly irrelevant sports facts was finely honed. Nearly 75% of the men surveyed were able to list the starting line-up for the '69 Mets. The other 25% were in Rotisserie baseball leagues, which had clouded their memory. Yet, 100% of these men were unaware of the date of their own anniversary.

Spousal Referral for Hearing Check

The last identifying feature of this disorder is that the spouse of the MMMLS victim always requires her husband to get a hearing check. Monroe & Miller (1961) found that in a survey of 10,000 couples, in 9,999 of the cases the wife had forced her husband to get his hearing checked (in the other case, the wife was deaf). It is significant that out of 9,999 hearing checks not one of the husbands had a detectable hearing loss.

Additional research by Jackson & Presley (1996) revealed that the highest incidence for spousal hearing referrals occurs during football season. Jackson & Presley labeled this unique aspect of MMMLS as Wasted Hearing Auditory Transduction (WHAT).

References

Anderson, L., & Reynolds, B., (1993) Marital Discord in the Garden of Eden, *Journal of Biblical Marriages*, Vol. 1, p. 1-2, 1993

Barr, R., & Arnold, T., White Trash Weddings
White Trash Quarterly, Vol. 202, p. 789-798, 1994
Fortensky, L., & Taylor, E., Why Men Don't Listen: It Could be MMMLS *Journal of Why Men Don't Listen*, Vol. 999, p. 888-889, 1996

Jackson, M., & Presley, L. M., Another Reason to Hate Football Season *Journal of Fed-Up Wives*, Vol. 333, p. 765-777, 1996

Johnson, D., & Griffith, M., No Cure in Sight for MMMLS
Journal of Perpetual Ignorance, Vol. 76, p. 666-667, 1977

Johnson, D., & Griffith, M., Still No Cure for MMMLS: A Repeat Study *Dysfunctional Family Journal*, Vol. 3, p. 1-9, 1995

Lovett, L., & Roberts, J., (1995). How to Have a Wedding Ceremony and Not End Up on "America's Funniest Home Weddings"
Journal of Tragic Weddings, Vol. 15, p. 82-100, 1995

Monroe, M., & DiMaggio, J., The Stupid Things Married Men Remember, *Journal of Why Men are Stupid*, Vol. 97, p. 2222-2224, 1954

Monroe, M., & Miller, A., Married Men Can Hear, No Matter What They Tell You, *How to Tell if Your Husband is Lying*, Vol. 129, p. 31-33, 1961

Presley, E., & Presley, P., Precursors to MMMLS
Journal of Divorce Precursors, Vol. 77, p. 57-78, 1973

Reynolds, D., & Fisher, E., Married Men and Memory: Oy! What a Mess! *Divorce, Memory & Alimony*, Vol. 5, p. 344-354, 1959

Trump, D., & Trump, I., Mnemonically Challenged Men: Does Divorce Always Follow? *Problems with Men*, Vol. 43, p. 34-45, 1990

Wyman, J., & Reagan, R., What Men Forget
Journal of Applied Marriage, Vol. 55, p. 76-77, 1949

Personals Ads from the Edge

- Minimalist seeks woman.

- Patriarch of up-and-coming religion seeks altar girl.

- Submissive male seeks dominant female with extensive knowledge of knots.

- Superboy seeks Clarke Kent. Come fly with me.

- Bitter, unsuccessful middle-aged loser wallowing in an unending sea of inert, drooping loneliness looking for 24-year-old, needy, leech-like, hanger-on to abuse with dull stories, tired sex and Herb Alpert albums. Baby, you are my Tijuana Taxi.

- There is a little place in the jumbled sock drawer of my heart where you match up all the pairs, throw out the ones with holes in them, and give me some of those neat dressy ones with the cool black and red geometrical designs.

- Three-toed mango peeler searching for wicked lesbian infielder. Like screaming and marking territory with urine? Let's make banana enchiladas together in my bathtub. You bring the salsa.

- Me — trying to sleep on the bus station bench, pleading with you to give me a cigarette.

  You — choking on my odor, tripping over your purse trying to get away; at the last moment, our eyes meeting. Yours were blue.

  Can I have that dollar?

It's All in the Genes

David J. Robinson, M.D.

Women are from Venus, men are just wrong. An explanation of this fundamental truth can be found by looking in our genes. A woman's genetic complement consists of two X chromosomes, a man's an X and Y. A view through a microscope reveals a picture something like this:

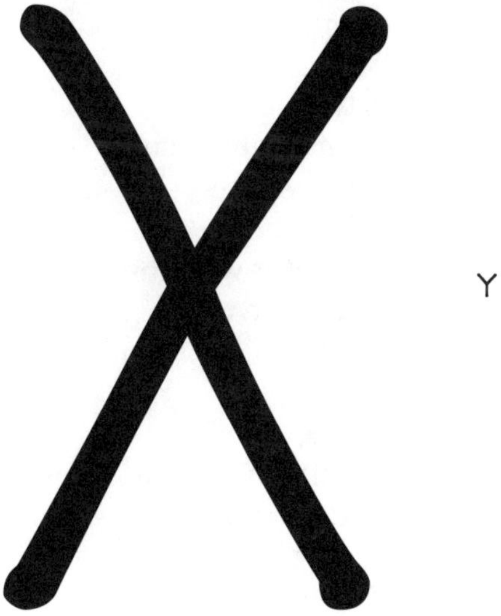

This illustration is drawn to approximately one-tenth the actual size difference between an X and Y chromosome.

Chromosomes make genes, which in turn make proteins that control bodily functions. This includes the ability to experience and perceive things beyond grunting as a social interaction. Women, with their vastly larger X chromosome, make oodles more proteins than do men. This results in the multi-layered, interactive biochemistry that makes up a woman's life. Men, on the other hand, get testosterone and perhaps one other mutant protein (whose function has yet to be ascertained) from the Y chromosome. Men are barely a step up from canines, their closest evolutionary buddies.

Things a Dog Wants to Do
- Sleep
- Eat
- Play
- Hump your leg
- Take a walk
- Drink water
- Run in packs
- Sniff fire hydrants
- Whine to get attention

Things a Man Wants To Do
- Sleep
- Eat
- Play sports
- Hump your friends
- Watch sports
- Drink beer
- Hang out with the guys
- Watch the news
- Whine to get attention
- Work

Women now have a scientific explanation for their frustrations with men and are encouraged to revise their expectations.

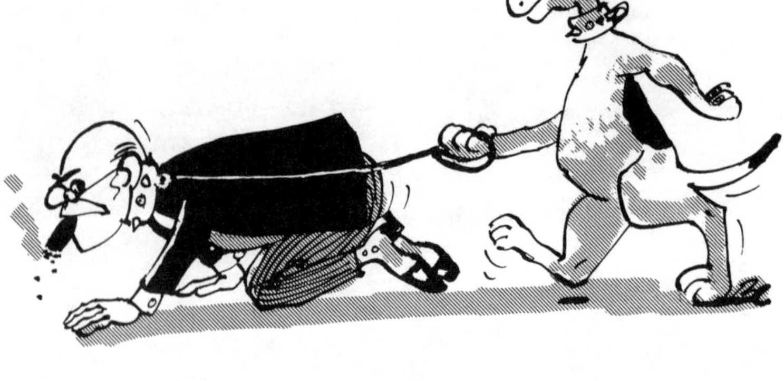

Chapter 6. Psych. Jokes

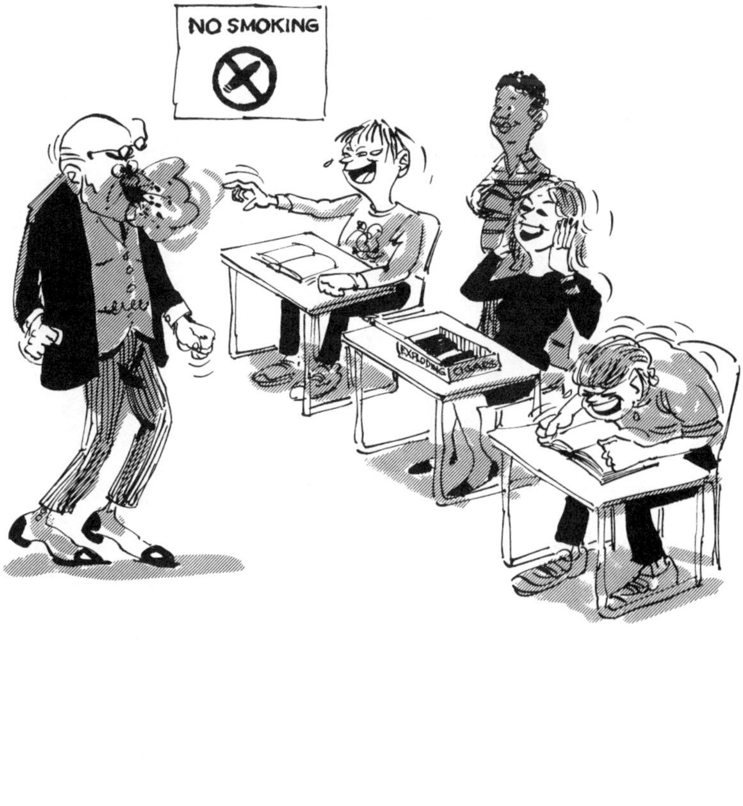

Psych. Jokes

A man is walking along the street. Suddenly, he is grabbed and pulled into an alley. After his assailants beat and rob him, he is barely able to crawl back to the street. As he lies there in a heap, a police officer passes him by. A troop of Boy Scouts does the same. Even a little old lady ignores him. Finally, a psychologist comes by and is shocked to find the man in such a condition. "My God!" he says, "Whoever did this to you really needs help!"

Sign on Pavlov's door — Please knock. DON'T RING THE BELL.

Secretary: Doctor, there's a woman here to see you who thinks she's invisible.
Psychologist: Tell her I can't see her right now.

I thought about doing a subliminal experiment, but just for a second.

Linda had been seeing an analyst to treat her fear that a monster was hiding under her bed. She hadn't had a good night's sleep in years and was becoming dismayed that her treatment was taking so long. In haste, she stops the analysis and consults another therapist. Three weeks later, she meets up with the original analyst. She looks ten years younger, feels well and is in the best mood she's been in for years.

"You look wonderful," says the analyst, "what happened since I last saw you?"

"I went to see a psychologist," she said enthusiastically, "and he cured my fears in one session."

"One session?" bemused the analyst, "how did he do that?"

"He's a behaviorist," she replied.

"A behaviorist!" exclaimed the analyst, "How did he cure you in one session?"

"Easy," she said, "he told me to cut the legs off my bed"

A psychiatrist is doing rounds on the inpatient ward. He notices that two patients are behaving in an odd fashion. The first man is sitting on the edge of his bed, with one hand on an imaginary steering wheel and the other on an imaginary gear shift. He is staring intently at the other end of the room and making loud noises like a race car.

"What are you doing?" asks the psychiatrist.

"I'm driving this Ferrari to New York" replies the patient.

Puzzled, the doctor moves on to the next bed where he sees some rhythmic activity going on underneath the covers. When he pulls the sheets back, he finds the second patient completely naked and lying face down on the mattress.

"And what are you doing?" asks the doctor.

"Well," replies the man, "while he's in New York, I'm having sex with his wife."

The doctor continues his morning rounds. This time he enters a room to see one patient sitting on the floor pretending to saw a piece of wood. The other patient is hanging from the ceiling by his feet.

"What are you doing?" asked the doctor.

"Isn't it obvious I'm sawing this wood in half?" replies the patient.

"OK. Can you tell me what your friend is doing?" asks the doctor.

"Oh, him. He thinks he's a light bulb." says the patient.

The doctor looks at the second patient and sees that his face is turning quite red.

The doctor asks the first patient, "Don't you think you should get him down from there — he looks like he might hurt himself."

The patient replies, "What?! And work in the dark?"

Definition of a psychologist: A man who, when an attractive woman walks in the room, turns to look at everyone else.

Patient: "Doctor, my wife thinks I'm crazy because I like sausages."
Psychiatrist: "Nonsense! I like sausages too."
Patient: "Good, you should come and see my collection. I've got hundreds of them."

Psychiatric Disorder Christmas Carols

- Cocaine Abuse — Ding Dong! Merrily on High!
- Delusional Jealousy — I Saw Mommy Kissing Santa Claus (And A Lot of Other Guys Too)
- Dementia — What Child Is This?
- Depression — God Rest, Ye Merry Gentlemen; Still, Still, Still; In The Bleak Midwinter
- Dissociative Fugue — Really Far Away in a Manger
- LSD Abuse — How Brightly Beams the Morning Star
- Mania — Deck the Halls and Walls and House and Lawn and Streets and Stores and Offices and Towns and. . .
- Multiple Personality Disorder — We Three Queens Disoriented Are
- Obsessive-Compulsive Disorder — Jingle Bell, Jingle Bell, Jingle Bell Rock, Jingle Bell, Jingle Bell, Jingle Bell Rock, Jingle Bell, Jingle Bell, Jingle Bell Rock, Jingle Bell, Jingle Bell, Jingle Bell Rock, Jingle Bell, Jingle Bell, Jingle Bell Rock
- Schizophrenia — Do You Hear What I Hear?

Personality Disorder Christmas Carols

- Antisocial Personality — A Fire Is Started in Bethlehem
- Avoidant Personality — Infant Holy, Infant Lowly
- Borderline Personality — You Better Watch Out, I'm Gonna Cry, I'm Gonna Pout, Then MAYBE I'll Tell You Why
- Dependent Personality — Rise Up, Sheep, and Follow
- Histrionic Personality — What Is This Fragrance So Appealing?
- Narcissistic Personality — Hark The Herald Angels Sing (About Me)
- Obsessive-Compulsive Personality — The Years Are Passing By (Get Busy)
- Paranoid Personality — Santa Claus is Coming To Get Me
- Passive-Aggressive Personality — On the First Day of Christmas My True Love Gave to Me (And Then Took It All Away)
- Schizoid Personality — Silent Night
- Schizotypal Personality — I Saw Three Ships

Where to Publish Your Paper

1. If you understand it and can prove it, then send it to a journal of mathematics.
2. If you understand it, but can't prove it, then send it to a physics journal.
3. If you can't understand it, but can prove it, then send it to an economics journal.
4. If you can neither understand it nor prove it, then send it to a psychology journal.

The aspiring psychiatrists were attending their first class on emotional extremes. "Just to establish some parameters" said the professor to the student from Arkansas, "What is the opposite of joy?"
"Sadness" said the student.
And the opposite of depression?" he asked of the young lady from Oklahoma.
"Elation" said she.
"And you sir" he said to the young man from Texas "how about the opposite of woe?"
The Texan replied "Sir, I believe that would be giddy-up."

A man runs to the psychiatrist and says "Doctor, you've got to help me. My wife thinks she's a chicken!"
The doctor asks, "How long has she had this condition?"
"Two years" says the man.
"Then why did it take you so long to come and see me?" asked the shrink.
The man shrugs his shoulders and replies, "We needed the eggs."

Chapter 7. Putting the "Psycho" back in Psychotherapy

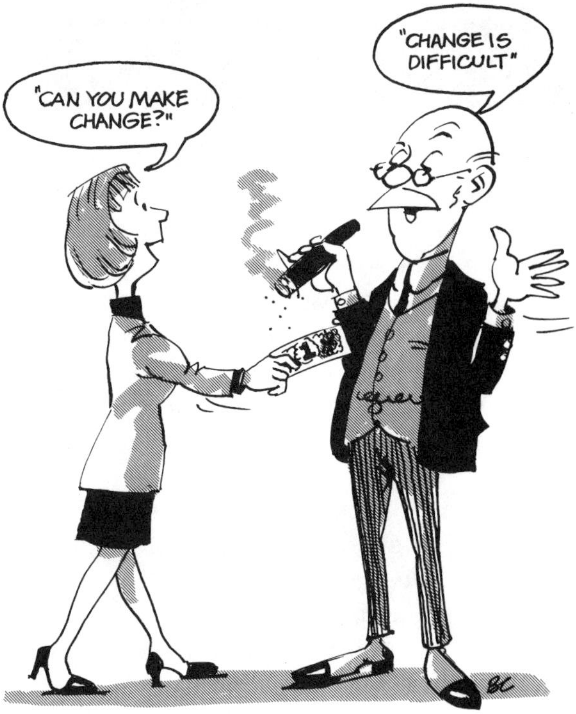

BCT: Blended Coffee Therapy

David J. Robinson, M.D.

It may look like an innocent concoction, but coffee has been a major force in shaping much of today's world. Next to oil, coffee is the world's most (legally) traded commodity, and a primary source of the world's most popular psychoactive substance — caffeine. As a crop, coffee conquered much of South and Central America, as well as making a significant impact in Ceylon, India, and Java. The bean has shaped laws and governments, exacerbated social inequities, caused the destruction of natural environments, and delayed the abolition of slavery. In no small way, coffee production continues to be a factor in the political conflicts in many countries to this day.

**Wherever the bean was ground,
civil unrest could be found.**

Wherever coffee has been introduced, it has caused revolution. It has been the world's most radical drink in that its function has always been to make people think. And when people think, they become dangerous to tyrants. The French and American revolutions were both planned in coffeehouses. In early 1676, King Charles II narrowly averted an uprising by aborting his ban on coffeehouses, as in his view they had become "the great resort of the idle and disaffected persons."

Coffee has had a long history of being a troublemaking social brew, even if the effects were not of revolutionary significance. Many rulers decided that people were having too much fun in coffeehouses. Patrons of such establishments have been accused of indulging in a variety of improper pastimes – ranging from gambling to irregular and criminally unorthodox sexual situations. Historically, lack of coffee was a sufficient enough basis for a Turkish wife to request a divorce.

> **"Coffee drunkards, as I may call them, are greatly increasing in number."**
> *Early 20th Century Physician*
> *London, England*

Medically, coffee has had a rather bipolar reputation. A detractor once said that it dried up cerebrospinal fluid and caused convulsions, which could lead to general exhaustion, paralysis, and impotence. Conversely, a proponent actually prescribed coffee because he thought that it sweetened the lower bowel and freshened the complexion.

The sexual effects of coffee have caused much heated debate. As early as 1674, women (who were banned from coffeehouses) published a petition claiming that coffee was turning their husbands into eunuchs, with nothing left stiff except their joints. As a rebuttal, the men of the time proclaimed that coffee made erections more vigorous, and added a certain "spiritual essence" to their sperm.

> **"Coffee is a grave menace to the health of the American people. It is a baneful drug that ought to be prohibited by law. Insanity has been traced to the coffee habit."**
> *Dr. John Harvey Kellogg*
> **(the cereal guy)**

The cognitive effects of coffee have been more clearly positive. Honoré de Balzac consumed pulverized, roasted grounds on an empty stomach, and had this to say of its effects: "Everything becomes agitated. Ideas quick-march into motion like battalions of a grand army to its legendary fighting ground, and the battle rages. Memories charge in, bright flags on high; the cavalry of metaphor deploys with a magnificent gallop."

Grounds For Treatment? A Modest Proposal. . .

Kaldi, the Abyssinian goatherd widely credited with discovering coffee beans, said (after eating some) that he felt he would never be tired or grouchy again. That coffee has revolutionary potential has been amply demonstrated. Harnessing the power of the bean is the next frontier in mental health. It is my opinion that many of the detrimental aspects of coffee have been due to improper preparation, ill-advised blends, or the use of adulterants.

Coffee, like the humors of ancient medicine, has four components: aroma, body, acidity, and flavor – much therapeutic value can be derived from balancing these components in a proper blend of coffee.

"The adulterations of coffee are so great that pure coffee is rarely to be had except in private families where the head of the house attends in person to preparation of the precious cup.
Coffee Drinker
New York City, 1872

Blend #1 — Treatment for Depression
"Cafe de Olla"
Place water, coarsely ground Mexican coffee, cinnamon, and brown sugar in a saucepan and bring to a boil. Reduce heat and simmer another three minutes. Use a fine strainer and serve in large, warm, heavy mugs (42 calories, 8g carbohydrate, 0g fat, 278mg caffeine).

Blend #2 — Treatment for Anxiety
"Mocha Mugs"
Stir cocoa and sugar together in a saucepan. Stir in

decaffeinated coffee and cold milk. When simmering, stir in vanilla. Ladle chocolate mixture into mugs, top with whip cream and then ground cinnamon (311 calories, 34g carbohydrate, 19g fat, 0mg caffeine).

Blend #3 — Augmenting Psychotherapy
"Spiced Viennese Coffee"
Place cinnamon sticks, cloves, and all-spice berries into an eight-cup carafe. Brew ground coffee according to the manufacturer's instructions. Allow coffee to steep for fifteen minutes. Strain into warmed coffee mugs, garnish with a sprinkle of cinnamon (17 calories, 1g carbohydrate, 1g fat, 121mg caffeine (using regular coffee)).

References

Mark Pendergrast
Uncommon Grounds
Basic Books, New York NY, 1999

Mary Ward
The Top 100 International Coffee Recipes
Lifetime Books, Hollywood FL, 1996

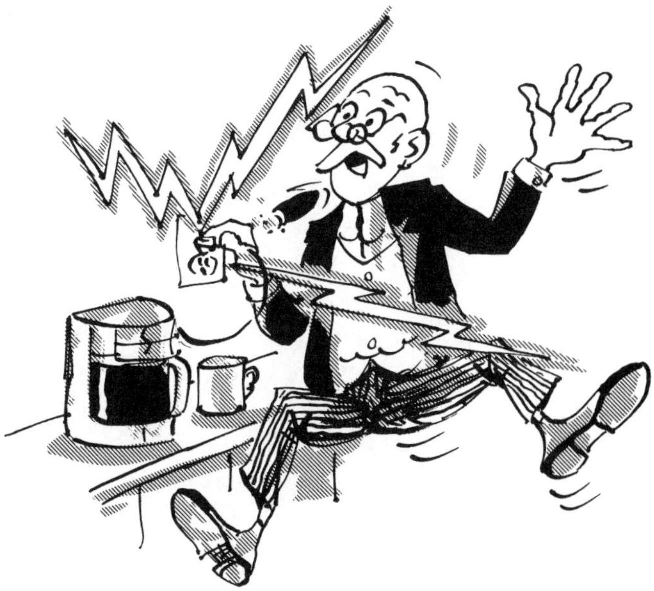

Past is prologue, and that's good enough . . .

Previous-Therapy Therapy

Michael F. Shaughnessy, Ph.D. & Tony Clifton
Portales, New Mexico

Recently, **Past-Life Therapy** (**PLT**) has become increasingly used as a treatment modality. Some skeptical scientists however, doubt that there is any empirical proof of a "past life" and insist that PLT is merely an artifact of therapeutic suggestion.

The first author concurs. The second author, since he is dead, does not. However, the point is that since there is no way to prove that a person has had a "past life," dealing with "past life issues" may not be productive. In order to deal with this problem, the authors have, however, recommended **Past-Therapy Therapy** (**PTT**) to resolve unresolved issues that may not have been completely worked out in previous therapy.

The theoretical construct is that many clients harbor ill feelings toward their past therapists. Some feel that they did not get their money's worth. Others did not like the chair or couch they were sitting on. Many resent the times of their appointments. Almost all patients have some unresolved issues with their past therapists.

In PTT, the sessions focus on the past therapist. If there are any current difficulties, they are blamed on the past therapist. If the client becomes litigious, the past therapist is the one who is sued. The use of the past therapist and an absent transference figure and target for flagrant projection can be a curative and lucrative factor in PTT.

Some people may block or resist PTT by indicating that they have never been in therapy. This too can be resolved. If a client cannot recall his or her past therapy sessions, this is clearly due to posttraumatic therapeutic amnesia (PTTA), and even more intensive attempts are made to deal with the past therapy.

The authors would also like to point out the protection afforded those who are paid a salary to engage in whimsical research. Since we are the ones who developed PTT and are its only practitioners, we will not have to suffer the indignity of having former patients enter into PTT with other therapists! QED.

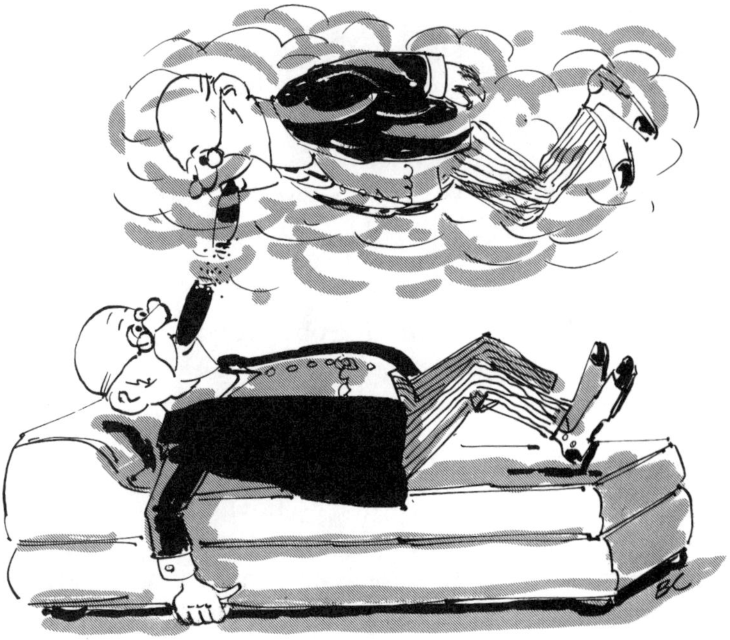

From the Therapist's Files

Larry Lister, D.S.W.
Kailua, Hawaii

Therapist: I'm glad we all have a chance to get together today. I'm sure you've been very unhappy Billy. Do you want to tell us about it?
Billy: No.
Therapist: Oh, I see. Well, I'm not sure I can blame you. It's hard saying things within the family sometimes.
Mother: I always say whatever I feel.
Therapist: You really get all your feelings right out there, huh? Do you want to tell us what you're feeling, then?
Mother: No.
Father: That's always the way. Yes and no. Yes and no.
Therapist: You mean you're saying your wife seems to give you double messages?
Father: No.
Therapist: You're saying no, she doesn't give you double messages?
Father: No.
Billy: Yes.
Therapist: That's an interesting observation, Billy. You seem to be contradicting what your father says. Do you often contradict him?
Billy: No.
Father: Yes.
Therapist: You mean, Father — now you see in family therapy we call people by their roles and that helps focus our interaction to the people whose interaction we are particularly focused on — so, now, you mean, Father, that Billy does contradict you?
Father: No.
Therapist: You mean 'no' he doesn't contradict you, or 'no'

he does contradict you?
Mother: Yes, he does.
Therapist: Now, Mother — you see, like father, we call you mother when we are referring to your role as mother. If we are referring to you in your role as wife, then we'll call you wife. So, then, to continue, Mother, are you saying 'yes' that your son does contradict his father or 'yes' that your husband means 'yes' to my question, or saying 'yes' as a way of speaking for your husband who you feel cannot speak up for himself?
Mother: No.
Billy: I think I may be getting confused.
Therapist: Good. Now we're getting at the heart of your conflict and beginning to uncover your basic schizophrenic adaptation. This is healthy and constructive and is, of course, our goal in family therapy. Now, then, Billy, are you saying you are confused because of the chaotic messages within the family, which leave you no out, save through disorganization, chaos, and nausea?
Billy: No.
Therapist: No, you are not confused and disorganized or 'no' you are not blaming your parents for subjecting you to their turmoil?
Father: I think I'm getting nausea myself.
Therapist: You feel ill?
Mother: This is making me sick.
Therapist: You feel ill?
Billy: I may throw up.
Therapist: You may?
Billy: I might.
Mother: Have the wish I wish tonight.
Father: Amen.
Therapist: You seem to be falling back on primitive socio-religious defenses. This is real progress. I'm really thrilled with the emerging dynamics here. There seems to be a core of chaos — a soft, gummy, loose, nexus holding this family structure together by but the frailest of tenuous threads.

Mother: I like to sew too.
Billy: Don't thread on me.
Father: A stitch in time is worth two in the bush.
Therapist: Marvelous! Marvelous! The dynamics are classic. You're even spouting your own proverbs. Does anyone like the one about the rolling stone?
Billy: I prefer the Beatles.
Mother: Well, give me Lawrence Welk anytime.
Father: I knew there was another man! I knew it! Who's this Lawrence person, anyway?
Therapist: Pure gold! Freud lives! This is so oedipal that I can hardly believe it! This whole shaky structure is woven around an oedipal conflict so profound in its implications that you, Billy, are just flipping out of your livin' gourd. Does anyone want to comment on this?
Mother: No comment.
Billy: Nolo contende. Nole contende.
Therapist: Now he's speaking in tongues. I think a conversion is around the corner for this family.
Mother: I'm getting kinda confused again.
Therapist: Of course! Of course! Why not, when you're all such a muddled mish-mash of primitive material which even Jay Haley will envy me forever because he'll be so jealous that he didn't get his hands on you.
Mother: But this all seems so different than I thought.
Therapist: What do you mean?
Mother: Well, we just came here with our son to work out a simple problem of whether he should join the school band or the track team. It just seems that this has gotten to be an awfully complicated discussion.
Therapist: So, who promised you a rose garden?
Father: I agree with mother — I mean, my wife. Everything seems so confused.
Therapist: But don't you feel purged? Like you're finally getting somewhere for the first time in the miserable existence of this family?
Mother: Not really. In fact, I've not really understood any-

thing that's been going on since we sat down here today.
Billy: Me neither.
Therapist: Now wait a minute. Who asked you? I think this had better be just between your parents and me, young man!
Father: Now, I think Billy's observations are important and, frankly, accurate.
Therapist: (testily) Well, if you're going to take his side then the hell with it. I thought we were all working together here but I can see this is just too pathological for family therapy. Frankly, I think I'd recommend a lobotomy for several of you, but that's up to the authorities.
Mother: (to the others) I think we'd better go. It seems we've not really gotten any place here today.
Father: Yes, I agree.
Billy: Me too.
Therapist: See, you're all in agreement. Isn't that terrific? You've just proved it. Family therapy really works!

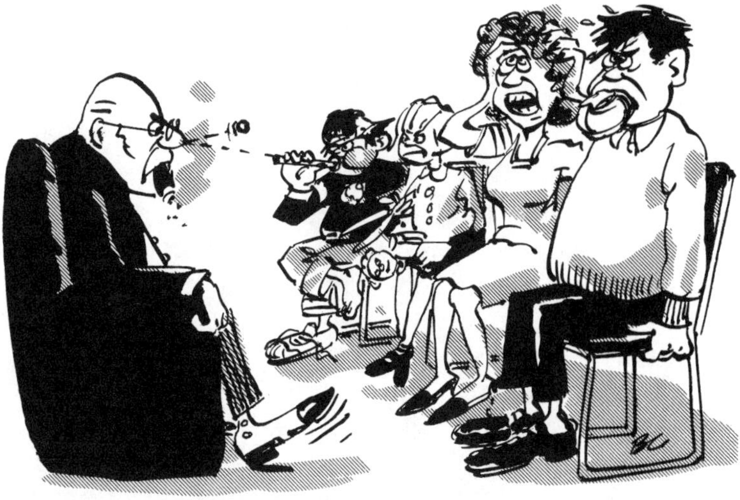

Sigmund Sez

David J. Robinson, M.D.

Learning how to be a good psychotherapist can be the most difficult six weeks of your career. Lacking from any current brand of therapy are the practical, face-saving maneuvers that conceal the fact that you weren't listening, attest to your brilliance, and keep patients coming back for more.

Example #1 — Change the Problem

Patient: "Doctor, I wonder if my lack of success in relationships is due to attachment issues from my childhood. After all, I was set adrift in a river and raised by alligators."
Sigmud Sez: "That's nonsense. Even gators love their young. What you haven't done is register with enough online dating services. Remember, you've got to tantalize potential mates by using romantic imagery. Plagiarize some poetry, maybe. Then try some of these websites:
www.loveamongthebullrushes.com
www.basketharmony.com
www.gatoromance.com

Example #2 — Postpone Your Comments

Patient: "This is the ninth week in a row that we've discussed my dream about drowning. Isn't it clear that this is an expression of my fear of commitment — getting in over my head — just like I'm drowning?"
Sigmund Sez: "Let's not rush things. First we need to explore your latent and manifest dream content in light of the day residue. Then you need to paint the images from your dream in art therapy, or better still, re-enact the whole dream in film therapy. After you take some swimming lessons and pass your boards in psychiatry, then maybe you can interpret your own dreams. For now, let's get back in the water."

Example #3 — Change Psychotherapy

Patient: "Is it possible that I had a dream about you drowning as a transference manifestation?"

Sigmund Sez: "Where is your homework? Did you construct your list about which fluids you are most fearful of me drowning in? Where is the rest of the group? Stop doing that! Was your last serum level in the therapeutic range?

Example #4 — Write a Book

Patient: "I just met someone I really like. I knew we were meant for each other when he said 'See you later, alligator' at the end of our first date. How do I stop myself from sabotaging this like all my other relationships?"

Sigmund Sez: "My book clearly says on page 296 that you are not supposed to ask your therapist direct questions."

Example #5 — Don't Give Advice

Patient: "All this insight is wonderful. I understand my problem from three theoretical orientations. But what do I do about it? How do I translate this knowledge in to action? I need some advice."

Sigmund Sez: "All this pleading reminds me of my formative years at the Jungerplatz Institute. There, I begged for advice. My supervisor told me that if you give a starving man a fish, you feed him for a day. If you teach him how to fish, he will learn to drink beer.

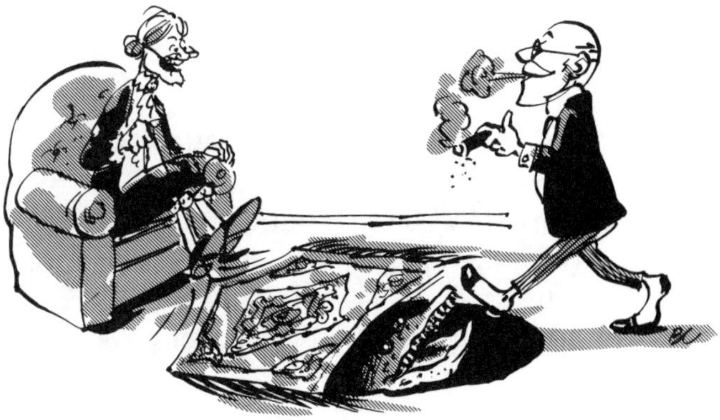

A Quick Cure for the Time-Obsessed

Joel Kirschbaum, Ph.D.
Hillsborough, New Jersey

This program replaces the traditional twelve step approach. Research has shown that time obsessed-patients feel there are up to six excessive steps, so they take them two at a time. To accommodate their haste, the program was severely shortened and speeded. The traditional apology step to those previously offended was deleted since this often reminds uncured time-compulsives of the origins of ancient, anger-inflaming, incidents. This fast, four-step regimen reduces rage, shrinks stress, and diminishes demeaning mutterings to the dawdling.

Group therapy is often a poor choice to treat time-compulsive patients since they always keep an eye out for each other's arrivals. Also, they often imitate each other's bad behaviors (e.g. if one patient sees a vehicle marked 4 x 4 and compulsively spray paints "=16" on the side of an SUV, then they will all start doing this). The downside to the therapist for facilitating a fast cure is that time-compulsive patients are punctual and pay promptly.

Step I.
Cope With Time Compulsion Using Technology

If you trapped in traffic, a time-utilizing tip is to use the ever-ready cell-phone to call, complain, and condemn. This is also an opportunity for therapists to sell cell-phone subscriptions featuring a multitude of minutes, as well as DVDs of Wagner's 14-hour ring cycle for portable players.

Step II:
Cope With Time Compulsion Using Internalized Diversions

This next step involves thinking and looking. For example, the patient could watch people at the post office as the line inches ahead as patrons hesitantly choose between different commemorative stamps to find the best color combination for each individual envelope. This allows the patient time to have a fantasy about someone else in line without exposure to communicable diseases or risking a significant other's wrath.

Step III.
Have the Patient Consider Lost Time to be an Investment

Divert attention of the time-compulsive from the delay itself by having the patient consider it as possible savings. This is via a proposed system of formal time-lost compensation wrung from the appropriate authorities. Here is how this kind of time-credit would work in a situation involving a wrong tax bill, which consumes 2 hours and 22 minutes of traumatic time to correct, via the telephone and various calling trees. Disconnects, misdirects, and repetitive music should result in triple time transfer credits. These 7 hours and 6 minutes of time credit should be cumulative, with the option of the holder using them to go to the front of post-office, customs, or other government lines. Such credits should also be sellable to individuals sentenced to prison, something like a "Get Out Of Jail Free" card. Anecdotal evidence indicates that authorities would accept and encourage such a system since uncured compulsives would hoard the credits anyway, rather than redeem them. Alternatively, encourage using the "dead" time to think of ways of getting even.

Step IV:
Provide the Perception of Power

Time anxiety can be reduced by having the therapist act to empower the patient. Suggest involvement in forming a local chapter of "The Rage Reduction Foundation," which would give time-compulsive patients a sense of control and influence while they are waiting. The Foundation would relieve patient stress by, for example, immediately towing illegally double-parked cars from, say, Philadelphia to Phoenix.

The author offers no compensation for time wasted reading this semi-autobiographical essay. It was written with the unintended assistance of an airline that had a six-hour flight delay due to pilot lateness (you know who you are and exactly what type of mail to expect) and Burger King, who supplied sustenance as well as the paper napkins used for writing paper. The purpose of my flight was to attend a Conference for Time-Compulsiveness. Although the sessions were scheduled to begin Monday at 9:00, since everyone was there by Friday night, meeting began immediately in order to end gratifyingly early.

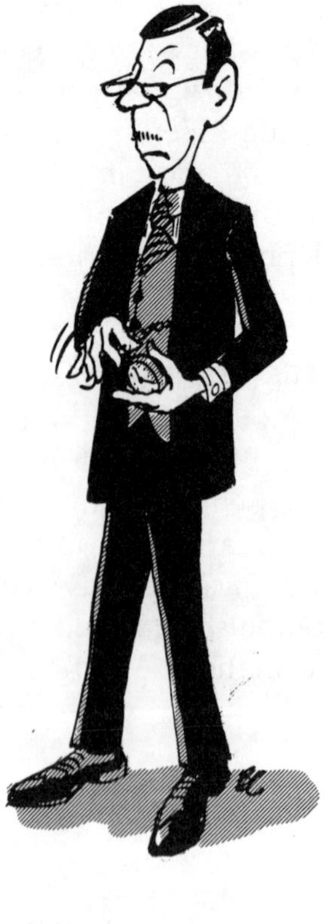

Gavin deRento, the world's most time-efficient human.

Chapter 8. Symptoms & Syndromes

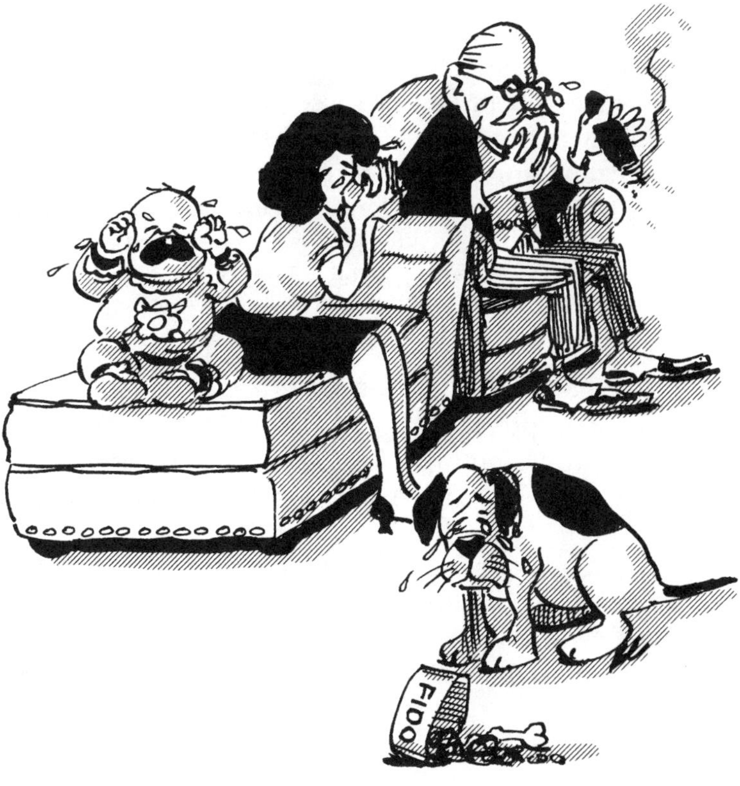

The Genetic Basis of Administosis

Stewart Cameron, M.D.

"I began to get suspicious when my husband said he was 'empowering the children to form a committee to create a family mission statement.' Then, last week, he told the dog and cat they had to 'pursue opportunities' outside our home because we were 'downsizing.' I decided to seek help from a physician after last night. My husband came to bed and announced that he 'wished to deploy our clinical thrusts in a strategic merger.' "

This unfortunate woman was the victim of a tragic disease; her physician husband had "gone into administration." The desire on the part of an otherwise normal clinician to assume bureaucratic responsibilities has always been considered a puzzling, and somewhat annoying, personality quirk. There is now sufficient evidence to propose that administrators are in fact genetically determined and are maladaptive homozygotes for an otherwise beneficial genetic mutation.

Diagnosis and Natural Course of Illness

Since it is now apparent that this state represents a true disease, I am proposing that physicians with managerial tendencies be considered to be suffering from administosis.

There is one major criterion for diagnosing the syndrome: the fixed delusion that the victim's organizational activities are somehow helpful, a misguided belief that persists in the absence of all validation and despite considerable evidence to the contrary. This state is pathognomonic. There are several minor criteria as well. The tendency to administer should be suspected when someone demonstrates:

- An obsessive desire to write and widely distribute their random thoughts (typically called memoranda)
- Compulsive use of voice mail (indeed, any doctor who actually uses the "distribution list" function should be considered affected unless proven otherwise)
- The hallucination that computers can make anything better
- A tendency to associate with other affected people in groups called committees
- The desire to force normal people to participate in the activity with them

All physicians are forced into some aspect of administration early in their careers. Typically they are assigned to hospital committees or managerial posts in their practices. Most survive using the time-honoured practice of truancy until they learn the art of total absenteeism.[1] However, a small number become enamoured of their administrative duties for reasons previously unexplained. They devote increasing amounts of time to governance to the detriment of their clinical skills (and incomes). In the most advanced stages, physicians suffering from administosis enter the final stages by seeking the elusive MBA.

Historical Theories

The condition of clinical administration has been known for millennia. (The term comes from the Latin roots *ad*, meaning toward, *mini*, meaning small or trivial, and *ration*, meaning portion, which literally translates as "working to give everyone something inconsequential.") Theories about why doctors take up administrative duties have varied through the ages. The ancient Egyptian physician, Amentrouble, believed that administrative jobs should be created to remove ineffective professionals from active duty. "Where a doctor has seen more floods of the Nile than he has teeth, he should stop reducing ruptures and begin to push papyrus instead," he wrote. Pharaohs in ancient Egypt were entombed with their chief administrators, as evidenced by the presence of hieroglyphic minutes-of-meeting documents and cuneiform quality-assurance reports found inside several pyramids. Initially it was presumed this practice was a sign of their importance to the deceased king. However several skeletons have recently been found inside the pyramid of Cheops clutching phoney agenda documents. It appears they had been lured inside for disposal, baited by the promise of a special committee meeting.[2]

We must blame the Greeks for advancing the concept that an administrative position is honourable. Hippocrates wrote, "Where a healer has cauterized a thousand haemorrhoids, it is a bad sign. He should lay down his poker and take up the stylus to better organize the performance of his younger colleagues." Remember, Hippocrates also thought that the arteries contained air. The great physician Galen felt that administrators were born, not made. He proposed that the condition was the result of an excess of the humors bile, phlegm and blood because of administrators' propensity to be simultaneously bilious, phlegmatic and sanguine. In a landmark 1899 monograph, Freud and colleague[3] proposed that administrative tendencies were the result of traumatic toilet training. They theorized that this was responsible for the preoccupation with performing ritualized ceremonial activities such as writing bylaws.

Some observers believe that clinical administrators are able to voluntarily control their activities, and therefore are guilty of a sin against nature. They have proposed that administrators "convert" to "normalcy," but this approach has proven dangerous.[4] More knowledgeable authorities accept that these people are indeed suffering from an illness. As Mungbean[5] wrote, "You have your every fault brought to your attention daily, and your judgement is constantly questioned. It's kind of like being the parent of teenagers. You become an administrator voluntarily only if you like to get beat up and make less money...sure, normal people want more of that!" Despite numerous attempts to free administrators of their own self-destructive tendencies, and to free the planet of administrators, they have persisted to modern times. Why has such an apparently maladaptive subset of the population survived? As I will show, it is because the gene that causes administrative behaviour confers an evolutionary advantage to heterozygotes.

Our team has discovered the locus of the administrator's gene using hospital management as a model for the condition. The isolation technique involved liquidization of tissue samples from several VPs of medicine, hospital chiefs and university department heads (a process that received surprisingly quick approval from our ethics board, who graciously suggested that we frappé a few specimens whole — unfortunately we could not find a blender large enough, although one nursing director offered to start a funding drive to buy one). We used molecular probes on the liquefied sample to look for the "bombastic" gene, which has been shown to be associated with the administosis gene.[6]

Our analysis shows that the administosis gene produces a recurrent translocation involving the ends of 2 acrocentric chromosomes, 14 and 21. In this previously undescribed process, 3 pieces of DNA were repeatedly exchanged in a recurring pattern between the 2 chromosomes.

Because having a single copy of the administrator mutation appears to confer the ability to simultaneously manage several different problems, we proposed the name "the juggle gene." This skill is highly respected in virtually all cultures, evidenced by the use of expressions "to keep all the balls in the air" and to "juggle one's responsibilities." While some manifestations of this ability are frowned upon (e.g., juggling the books), the trait is generally regarded as necessary for professional success. Alas, some people receive 2 copies of the allele, making them compulsive pushers of paper and victims of the administosis syndrome.

Therapy

Because it is genetically based, the state is presently incurable.

Those afflicted should be treated with benevolence and reassured that their work is valuable. However, under no circumstances should their delusional plans actually be followed, lest grief befall all concerned. The best we can provide is sympathy to the family members and grief counselling to medical colleagues. There are some online self help discussion groups devoted to this topic (e.g., alt.admin.recovery), but most of the users are the sort of people who accept advice from total strangers over the Internet.[7]

References

1. The memoranda of Machiavelli, with special emphasis on "while you were out" notes. *Archives 'R' Us* 1995;677:612-7.

2. Callipygous A. *Administration's place in history*. New York: Colonphon Publishers; 1996. p. 145.

3. Freud S, Jurgen Regrethat. *Die Analretentivedummkopfen*. Vienna: Uberallesbuchen; 1899. p. 67.

4. Nutzoi D, B Onkers. Hyper-analysis of 36 meta-analyses of executive voice mail greetings. *Administrivia Ad Infinitum* 1997;46:13356-60.

5. Mungbean R. *The commercialization of morality — from Socrates to Big Soren K's deontology barn*. Stockholm: House O' Ethics Publishing; 1998. p. 123.

6. Vapid R. Restriction fragment length polymorphism in bureaucratic twits. *Recreational Genetics* 1997;6:32-67.

7. www.borneveryminute.com/credulous/glaikit.html.

Reprinted with permission of the Canadian Medical Association Journal.
This article was originally published in:
CMAJ • DEC. 15, 1998; 159 (12) 1467 — 1468

False Malingering Syndrome

Steven Rothke, Ph.D.
Northbrook, Illinois

A major lament of defense attorneys has been the inability to distinguish real malingering from its exaggerated forms. False Malingering Syndrome (FMS) was believed to begin when college students were asked to feign a malingered presentation of a known disorder. Perhaps due to a failure to debrief these subjects, they continue to simulate malingered presentations, likely in anticipation of a $10 payoff for 30 minutes of their time. Some of the subjects eventually sustained real injuries, and appeared for an independent psychological exam. The poor defense expert is then faced with the moral dilemma of whether he should lie and call the person a genuine malingerer, or tell the truth and label the person as having FMS. The author has developed a screening test, the Feigning-it-Loving-it-And-Knowing-it-Examination (FLAKE) to assist with this problem.

F.L.A.K.E.

- I would never take advantage of someone without a good incentive.

- Thoughts never occur to me.

- I experience more pain when asleep than awake.

- Elvis was greater than the Beatles.

- I have never taken a psychological test that I didn't like.

- A missed diagnosis is a missed opportunity.

- My father was a man.
- I would like the work of a neurolawyer.
- I sometimes feel as if my ears were switched at birth.
- Someday my syndrome will develop into an actual disorder.
- Following my injury, I could no longer recall my past lives.
- It is impossible to catch a sexually transmitted disease by suing someone.
- My injury would never have occurred if I didn't have good insurance coverage.
- There has been an increasing numbness behind my nose.

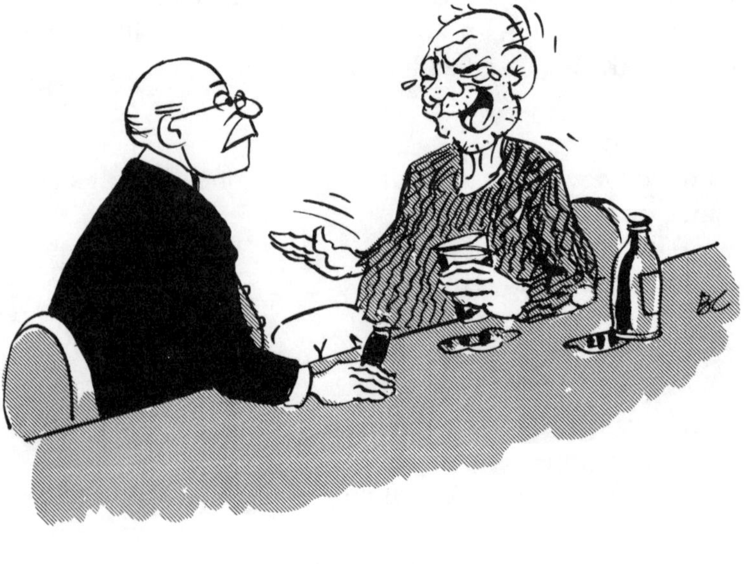

Trek-ATalk-AMania

Ronald H. Rozensky, Ph.D.
Evanston, Illinois

Early and unpublished letters written between Freud and science fiction author Jules Verne were recently compiled by Nemo and Fogg (1993). These letters first highlighted the tendency for metaphorical communication based upon self immersion within a fantasied story line. Originally referred to as *halodeckatropia* (Troi, stardate (sd. 2459), or *halosphereism* in its autoerotic form (Quark, sd. 2198), this phenomena has exploded in popularity since the 1960's and has been classified in the Diagnostic & Startistical Manual (DSPM) as **Trek-ATalk-AMania** (TAA). TAA is described as the increasing tendency to refer to the events in one's own life to the characters and concepts from the various Star Trek television episodes and movies.

Diagnostic Nosology

The current nosology detailing TAA (McCoy, Crusher, Bashir and Troi, sd. 2395) highlights three levels of psychopathology. **a**-TAA disorder is seen in those who make only passing references to television-based science fiction. This is a subclinical syndrome often seen in either the feeble minded or those unaware of their own surroundings. Those diagnosed with **b**-TAA become agitated when they miss an episode of Star Trek and resort to repeated, self-administered doses of video-taped episodes. **b**-TAA sufferers reference major life events to Star Trek or some other popular science fiction genre, however they are aware of the analog nature of their own experiences. **c**-TAA is easily recognized in those who festoon their automobiles with window decals or bumper stickers stating, *Klingon War Academy*, *I Have a Child at the Vulcan Science Academy*, or *Ferengi Business School Grad.*

Repeated reference to themselves as characters within Star Trek has been noted in the **c**-TAA types (Kirk, Picard & Cisco sd. 2949). Further, these individuals require increasing dosages of science fiction in order to feel satiated (Dax, Data & Odo, sd. 2114; Troi & Riker, sd. 3401). Others have noted that the **c**'s tend to be overly computer literate and display some signs of *hackeroparallelism* (La Forge, O'Brien, and the other Dax, sd. 4199).

When questioned about the relevance of their obsession with these "future-oriented images" **c**'s can become self righteous (Riker & Stewart, sd. 2019), belligerent (Worf & Yar, sd. 2289; Nerys, sd. 2290), or superfluously analytical (Spock & Data, sd. 2109). In the florid state, there is a tendency toward extreme narcissism or omnipotence ("Q-ism"; Q, sd. 9999) or a reliving of the past and future simultaneously (Guinan, sd. 1999). One author has noted with concern that **c**'s lack financial responsibility (Quark, sd. 2113). Early *weslycrusherism* is pathognomonic in children and should be ruled out in cases where IQ is above 124. In adolescents, a tendency to blindly follow others in group or pack-like behavior has been noted (Borg, sd. 0000). Collecting of future-oriented memorabilia has been documented (Trekkie, 1968, 1989, 1993, 1997)

Treatment Recommendations

There are three treatments presently recognized for TAA — biological, psychotherapeutic, and self-help. Biologically, many investigators have focused upon the malignant properties of the little-studied tribble cell and the effects on cortical and subcortical aspects of brain (Bones, sd. 2459). The most common biological treatment for this disorder, however, focuses upon lithium treatment. Dilithium crystals have been known to have a warping effect on the "gabby" cells, resulting in less maniacal, analytical and scientific references. The mechanism of this psychopharmacological treatment is not presently known (Crusher, Scott & Amundsen, 1909). Occasionally pressing a small beeping box with flashing lights against the patients temple (unilateral) or temples (bilateral) will cause a slowing of the syndrome. (Dr. Who, 1967, 1972, 1982, 1988, and sd. 3429).

Psychotherapeutic treatments have included:

- *Implosion Treatment*: a rapid repeating of episode themes in close proximity to a black hole (Troi, sd. 2123)
- *Exposure Therapy*: continued viewing of a single, early, overacted episode near a source of Thalean radiation (Kirk, 1968)
- *Reflective Therapy*: a sci-fi knock-off of Gestalt therapy seen in a New Generation episode wherein the patient talks with various segments of his or her personality (Riker, sd. 2137)
- *Managed Care*: viewing an exciting episode in a limited or diminishing time period with important scenes deleted

Explorations into the relevance of managed competition (Quark & Hillary, 1994) is still in the experimental phase. Cognitive and psychoanalytic treatments have been found to have a similar basis (Spock & Data, sd. 2120) because they both ignore the concept of free will (Borg, sd. 2013). However, both are favored compared to humanistic treatments (Carl Rogers, Mr. Rogers, Will Rogers & Free Willy, 1992) because many who suffer from TAA are not humanoid. Psychoanalytic references to the id, ego and superego being represented by Captain Kirk, Dr. McCoy and Mr. Spock, (respectively) indicate the terminal phase of TAA where treatment is no longer recommended.

The self help movement, TAA-Anonymous (TAAA) is a 1200-step program based upon admitting ones powerlessness over the collective (Borg, sd. 2013b) and reaching for a higher power (Aliens on Cardassia 12). Herein, one must make amends for the numerous sitcoms, dramas, and sporting events missed whilst compulsively revisiting old reruns (La Forge, "On the holodeck, sd. 2338). Accepting the adage, "one episode, then hooked" (Vulcan, sd. 2121) has been found therapeutic. Finally, realizing that trek-amania is the video experience of choice (Skywalker, Solo, and Obiwan, 1978) will help the victim avoid relapse (DS9, StarTrek: The Next Movie, 199?).

Conclusion

TAA is a recurring disorder that takes one where no one has gone before. Its five year (old strain) to seven year (new strain) duration forces those so afflicted to explore strange new worlds of self absorption. Treatment often involves boldly going forward without the camaraderie and small talk inherent in the addiction to metaphorical references to life in a future where, curiously, all creatures are bipedal and speak English.

batlh Daqawlu'taH (Worf and Okrand, 1992).
ghltlh vlghltlta'bogh DalaD'a' (Worf and Rozensky, 1993).
jiHtaHbogh noDev vlSovbe'. naDevvo' ylghoS.

References

Okrand, M., **The Klingon Dictionary**
New York: Pocket Books, 1992

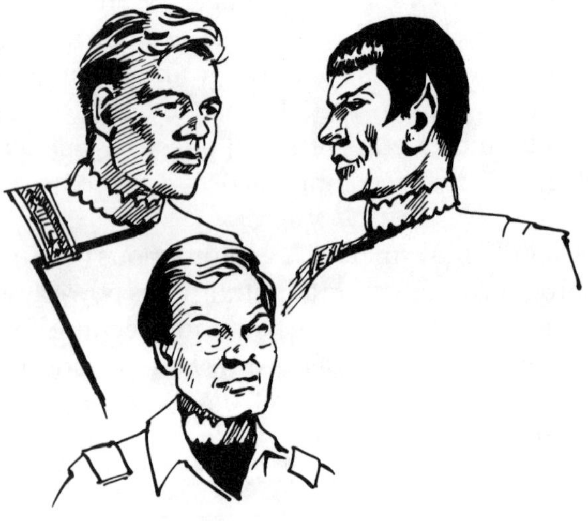

From Dystrepidatio to More Effective Worrying

Rudolph Philipp, Ph.D.
Toronto, Ontario

The core concept of **dystrepidatio** is that individuals worry themselves sick about things that generally don't happen. In the majority of cases, the neurotic energy wasted on worrying about the wrong things prevents sufferers from responding to genuine worries when disruptive events actually occur (and are invariably things the person failed to worry about).

Dystrepidatio is the diagnosis assigned to those who *realize that they worry about the wrong things and now worry that they don't know what they should be worrying about.* Mental health professionals have ignored this syndrome for too long, as evidenced by the absence of dystrepidatio from the DSM. This article presents a comprehensive overview of this important condition.

The word worry comes from the old English "wrygan" and from the German word "wurgen" or to strangle (Von Bulow, 1979). It is unclear whether this indicates that worry has the potential to strangle someone, or describes the urge to strangle the person causing the worry. The term "worry wart" has been in common usage for much longer than empirical studies have been carried out. Attempts by a Hungarian physician, (Aggodik, 1950) to treat worry warts with "Compound W" yielded results which have mysteriously disappeared.

Tsouris and Tsouris (1988) cite cases where death may have

occurred from excessive worry. In retrospect, these patients may have been more accurately diagnosed as having other conditions (Kvetch, 1995). Research has shown that early recognition and intervention (Sublingual, 1978) can prevent the morbidity and mortality due to acute dystrepidatio. However, funding cutbacks are causing worries for worry researchers (AppréHension, 1990).

Frequently, governments have been criticized for maintaining statistics on the incidence and prevalence of alcoholism, suicides, kleptomania, etc., yet failing to worry about worriers. One explanation that has been offered is that since the majority of the population worries, counting all such cases would indicate that an epidemic was present, which would in turn be a cause for grave concern (Tracasser & Ennui, 1989).

Behavioral scientists have not yet adequately studied worrying, even though most people worry, and many seek counseling. Only one individual (Alfred E. Neuman, the gap-toothed dude from Mad Magazine) has ever publicly denied worrying on a repeated basis. Neuman has made a lucrative career out of challenging the beliefs of others that he is indeed worrying.

Worrying is considered an expectation of being a parent, however few are ever told how much is enough. A faculty member worried about tenure could get a real career boost by developing an instrument to measure the optimal level of worry, which presents the following possible clinical pictures:

1. Patients with too few worries will be told that they are not in the optimal range, and are therefore "abnormal." This will give more to worry about, and move them into the ideal range. Of necessity, they will need guidance on which new worries to have.

2. Patients having an optimal amount of worry will be told that they are in the normal range, and have nothing to worry about. This in turn will drop their total amount of worry and they will repeat the cycle in (1) above. Such patients are likely to require counseling on which worries they should now abandon.

3. Patients with an above-average amount of worry will be told so, further increasing their worrying. This forces them to decide whether they should devote more energy to their original worries, or whether they should start worrying about their worrying.

The Treatment of Dystrepadatio

As with all interventions, timing is important. Competent professional counseling is clearly needed to facilitate more effective worrying. Many people remain burdened with outdated worries ("Without a tan I'll look like a techno-dweeb) and would benefit if more contemporary worries were substituted ("If I get too much sun, I'll look like I have to work for a living"). Most people would prefer having hip concerns, and would gladly pay to avoid being ridiculed for having passé worries.

Developmental Considerations

Infants don't worry because they have as yet not developed the concept of a dry diaper, let alone a notion of the future (Sansouci, 1974). It would appear that parents aren't yet teaching their suckling infants how to worry effectively.

Case Example

A mother sat up late one night waiting and worrying about her teenage son who had not yet returned. Her other son suggested that she could go to sleep and he would wait up for his brother. Her reply was, "What good would that do? You don't know how to worry!"

Comment: If parents don't teach their children or give them opportunities, how will they learn to worry effectively? This woman could easily have given this responsibility to her son and gone off to bed. After a good night's rest, she could have asked him how his worrying went and praise any success that he may have had.

Other Therapies

In recent years, the phrase *Don't Worry, Be Happy* has been popularized. If people actually listened to this, few clinicians would still be in business. Such an event could devastate the sale of anxiety-reducing medication. It has been rumored that various pharmaceutical companies are bombarding the popular media with a subliminal variant.

Don't Worry, Be Happy **<<-->>** ***Don't Be Happy, Worry***

Summary

Worry needs to be recognized and given a true diagnostic label when it is dysfunctional. With proper funding for research, those suffering from dystrepidatio will be able to discuss their condition openly at cocktail parties. Until then, self-help groups initiated by ex-worriers can help support sufferers of dystrepidatio to cope more effectively with day-to-day worrying.

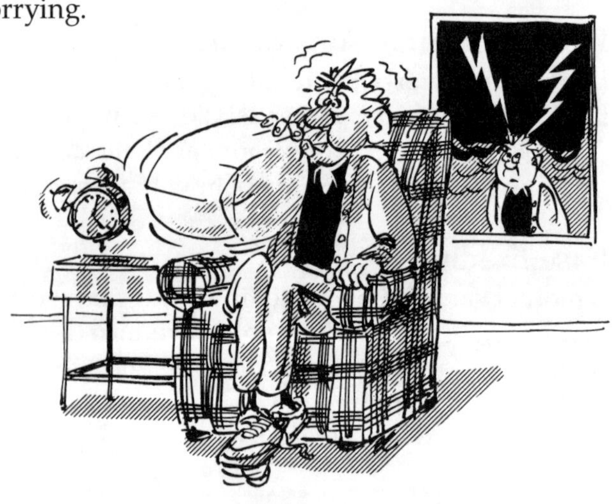

A Hidden Epidemic:
Post-Convention Stress Disorder

Sheldon F. Crusty, Ph.D., Terry Campbellson, Ph.D., Elmo Goldspoon, M.D., & Dilbert Binswanger, Ph.D.
Department of Psychiatry, Happyview Hospital

Authorities on traumatology, such as Bessel van der Kolk, Alexander McFarland, and Sheldon F. Crusty, have long observed a type of amnesia in the psychiatric profession regarding traumatic stress reactions. The events of World Wars I and II, for example, led to the widespread recognition of a syndrome known as "shell shock" or "soldier's heart," later known as posttraumatic stress disorder (**PTSD**). After World War II the syndrome was largely forgotten by psychiatrists. It was not until the Vietnam conflict that PTSD was rediscovered by the psychiatric community and reintroduced into the psychiatric nomenclature.

A similar professional amnesia has occurred for another disorder, described here for the first time. This disorder, called Post-Convention Stress Disorder (**PCSD**), is a widespread affliction of habitual attendees at academic conferences. Conferees typically recognize the symptoms of PCSD during and shortly after their attendance at conferences, often accompanied by vows to "dry out and never attend another conference again." Yet, just as PTSD was forgotten after World War II, conferees typically forget (repress?) the traumatic events associated with PCSD, only to sign themselves up for another poster session in Chicago.

The purpose of this article is to describe and illustrate the symptoms of PCSD. We do so in the hope that sufferers, suffering significant others, and health care professionals can better identify this often unrecognized disorder. We also share with readers some of our recent findings on the treatment of PCSD.

Symptoms of PCSD

According to criteria outlined in the 5th edition of Crusty's Compendium of Gratuitous Descriptions of Colleagues (**CCOGDOC**), PCSD is defined by a set of characteristic symptoms arising after attendance at one or more academic conferences:

1. **Hyperarousal**. This includes sweating, nausea, palpitations, and "feeling shaky." The symptoms are typically associated with feelings of dehydration and cravings for pizza and reprints.

2. **Dissociative Symptoms**. These are difficult for sufferers to describe, and are best illustrated by the following examples: (a) waking up in your Acapulco hotel room in wet clothes reeking of chlorine, (b) finding your mini-bar inexplicably depleted of beverages, (c) loss of shoes, and (d) inexplicably losing your overheads for the talk the next day. Typically, the latter occurs while "rehearsing" one's talk during all-night hotel room parties.

Examples of other dissociative symptoms were described by Dr. Goldspoon in 1978 after his first major academic presentation. He has probably forgotten these events, although his account merits recounting because of its historical interest:

"While attending a plenary talk, I realized I was wearing a name badge that said 'Helga' and then was surprised to find I was also wearing her clothes. Later, while unpacking my suitcase post-conference, I was hard-pressed to explain to my wife where I acquired the garter belt and exotic undergarments packed in along with the conference proceedings. She was not convinced by my confabulation regarding Eli

Lilly's discovery that free pens are no longer in vogue, and that the undergarments are a new line of promotional advertising. The fact that the garter was marked 'Helga' and not 'Eli' or 'Lilly' did not help matters either."

3. **Re-experiencing**. Some sufferers, particularly those with acute PCSD, complain of "flashbacks." Typically, these disturbing experiences are triggered by remarks made by other conferees, such as "Do you remember the crack you made about Francine's décolletage?" or "Do you remember what you did in the hotel pool last night?" Experts believe that statements such as these sometimes produce a form of false memory syndrome (**FMS**). Indeed, many sufferers of PCSD believe they are victims of FMS.

4. **Avoidance**. PCSD sufferers typically avoid activities that unduly deplete their already compromised cognitive resources. Thus, they avoid attending symposia laden with graphs, statistics, and the like. PCSD is associated with significant impairment in social and occupational functioning. PCSD sufferers are at heightened risk for getting their faces slapped during gala dinners, and for being photographed while doing the Macarena. These events can lead to loss of job opportunities, divorce, and other hardships. Loss of wallets, luggage, and speaker's notes are also common complications.

Conferees with chronic PCSD can be readily spotted. Aside from predilections for acronyms and spanking, they tend to give the same talk at conferences year after year. They also rely heavily on technical aids, in the hope of using audiovisual pyrotechnics to distract the audience from the meager content of their talks. Often the technology goes awry, and much of the talk is devoted to apologies about failed equipment. Chronic PCSD speakers often wax lyrical about how wonderful their talk would have been were it not for the technical glitches. Sometimes their apologetic blather is eloquent and entertaining; a welcome relief from dreary stuff they would have otherwise presented.

Symposium discussants with chronic PCSD also can be easily identified. They usually admit to having not read the symposium papers, often blaming gypsies for stealing the valued documents. PCSD discussants also have a tendency to snore throughout other speakers' presentations. This could be a dissociative defense or perhaps simply the effects of the night before. Some claim that their dreams provide valuable insights into the symposium topic but hasten to add that technological glitches prevent them from preparing slides or handouts to convey their valuable discoveries.

The Need for Further Research

As critics have rightly noted, the literature to date on PCSD is highly anecdotal, often collected in hotel bars or washrooms. Now is the time for large scale epidemiologic studies. To advance our understanding of this affliction, we have submitted a multi-million dollar grant to the National Institutes of Health. We have been informed that the reviewers will examine our submission just as soon as they've "slept it off." We assume they're referring to the devastating effects of PCSD. Another important avenue for further research is to identify protective factors. Recent reports suggest that PCSD is particularly rare at Mormon conventions. Some scientists suggest that Mormons may carry a PCSD-protective gene. Others argue that polygamy confers protection against PCSD. Sociologists point to the absence of mini-bars at Mormon conventions.

Treatment

With regard to treating the effects of PCSD, so far all we have are anecdotal reports from humanitarian aid workers. Reports suggest that Eye Movement Desensitization and Reprocessing (EMDR) is effective but difficult for patients to tolerate. Apparently, the waving of the therapist's hand pro-

duces unpleasant side effects such as nausea and vomiting. Rational self-statements appear to be of limited value. Tylenol coma therapy appears promising, particularly for sufferers who don't have an early morning flight
the next day.

For those PCSD sufferers who need to remain at least semi-alert (i.e., those who have give a talk), vodka martini therapy (VMT) appears to be the treatment of choice. Flipper Pharmaceuticals — makers of the Zoloft/ Rogain/Viagra drug cocktail for bald patients with sexual obsessions — are currently looking into the possibility of marketing VMT in capsule form. We look forward to the availability of this important treatment in a mini-bar near you. In the mean time, PCSD sufferers are encouraged to partake of services available from the masseuses at the Flipper convention booths.

By Steven Taylor, Ph.D.
Vancouver, British Columbia

Post-Dramatic Dress Disorder

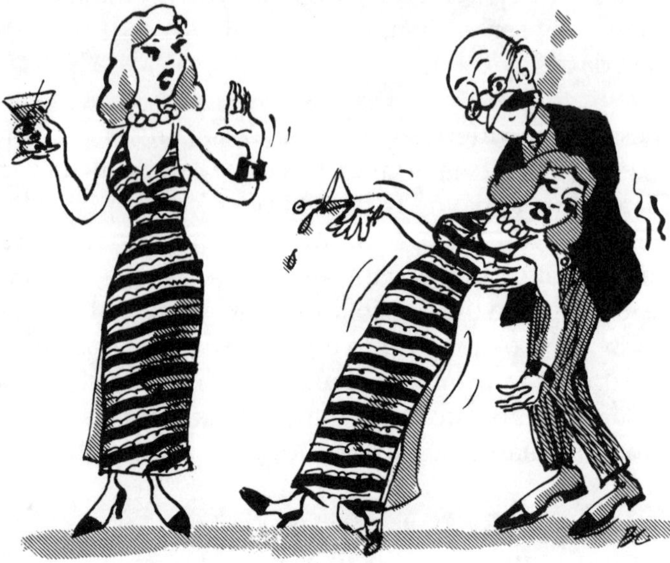

Anoxia Nervosa

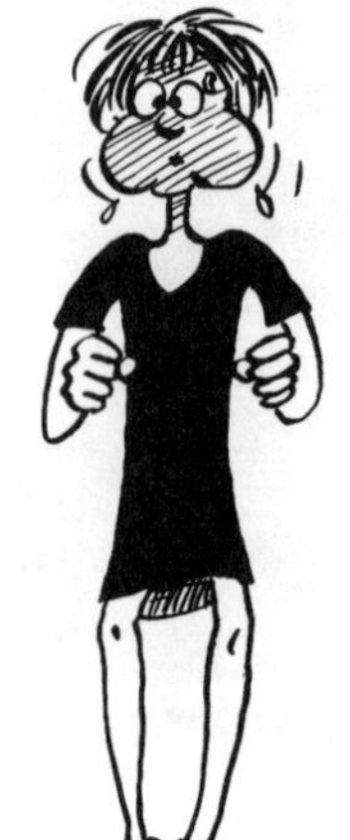

Chapter 9.
The
Artery

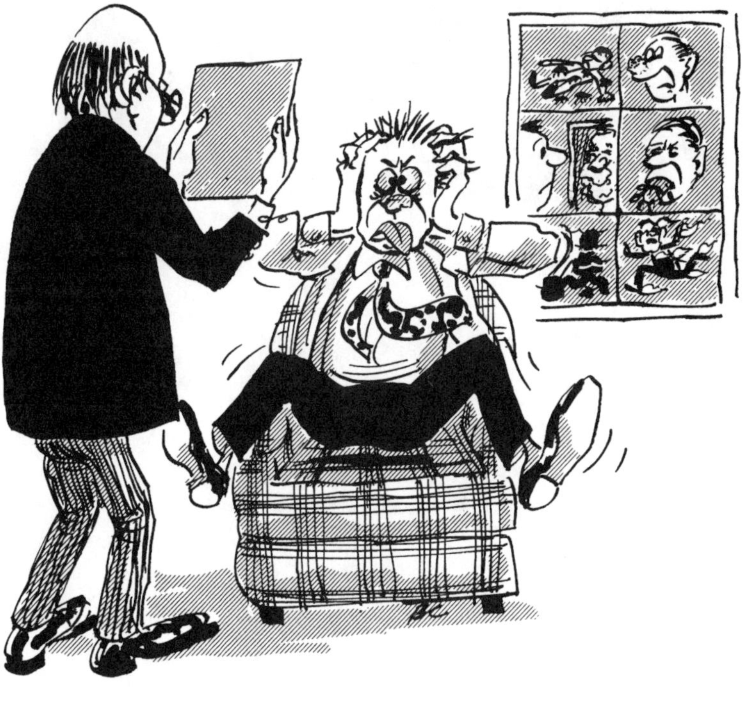

The "Rorshock"

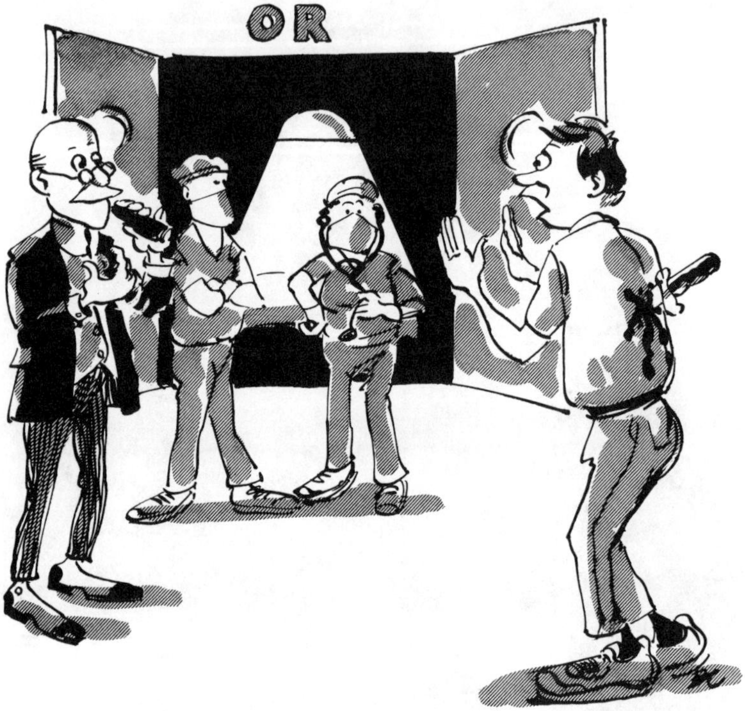

"The surgeons are here to take out the knife.
I am here to solve the real problem."

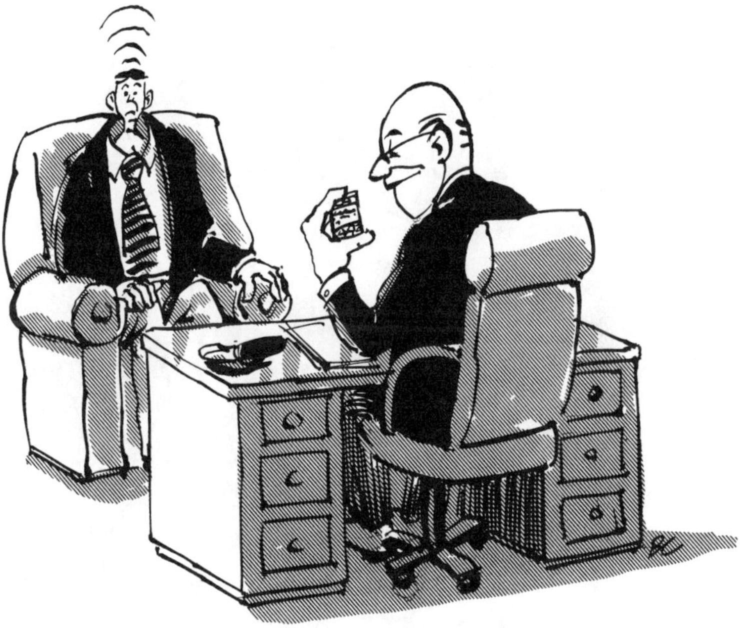

"Funny, this usually happens with psychotherapy."

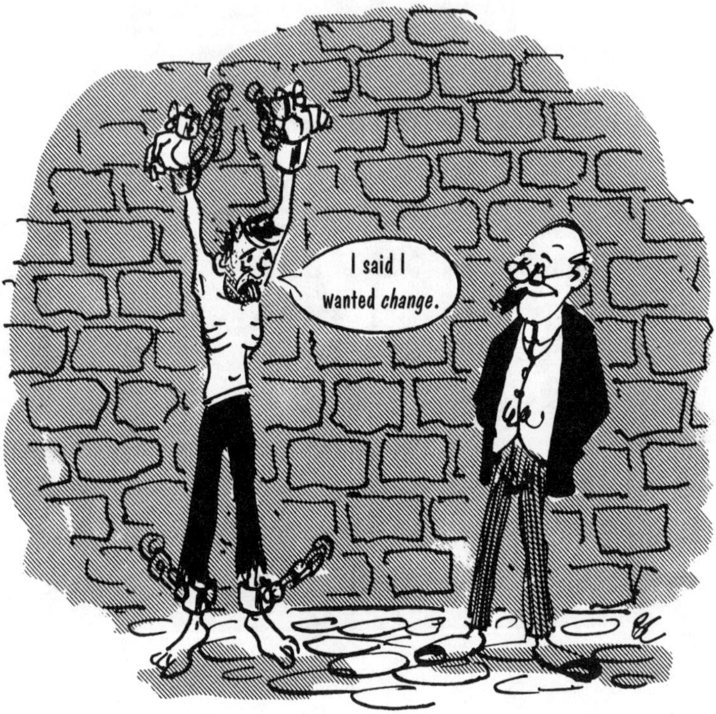
I said I
wanted *change*.

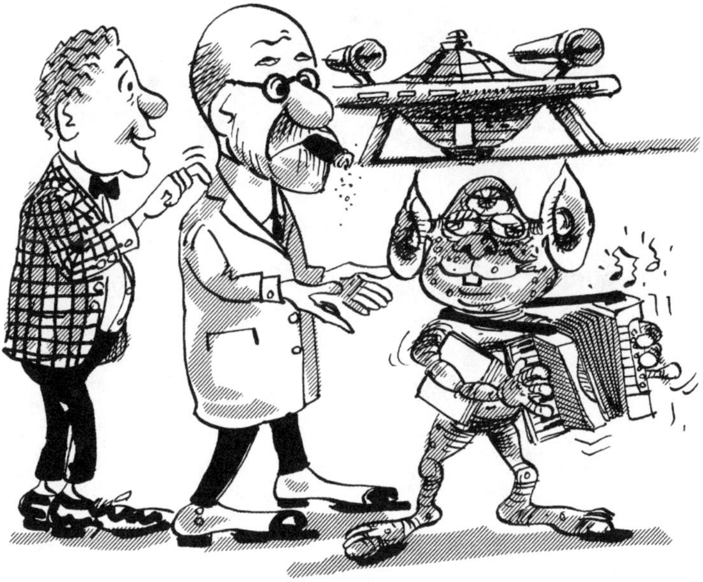

"We haven't seen one around here for a while either.
Apparently they're called 'Neo-Freudians'
or something like that."

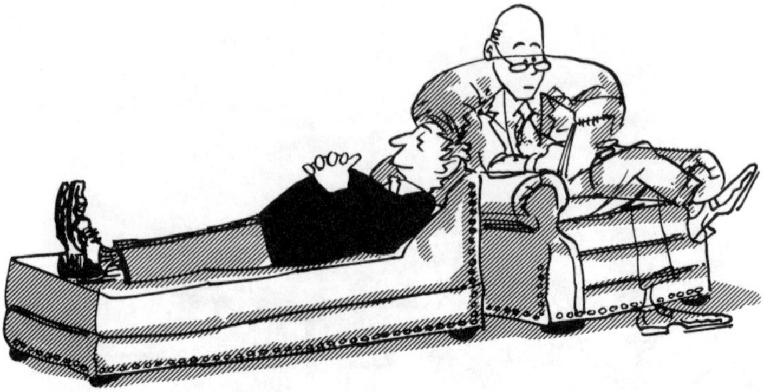

"I had been seeing a therapist for three years. . .

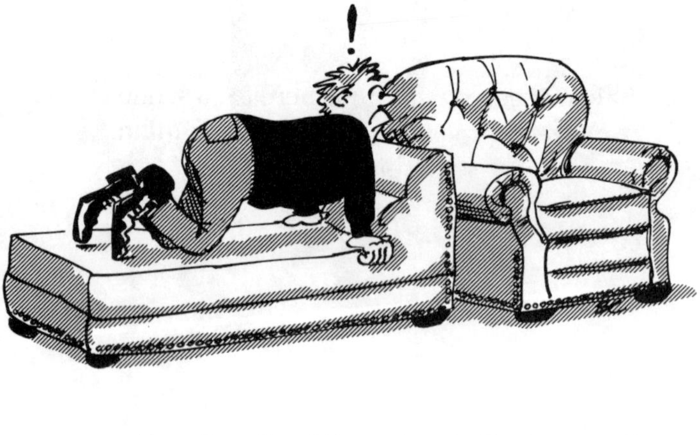

. . .then I realized I was just hallucinating!"

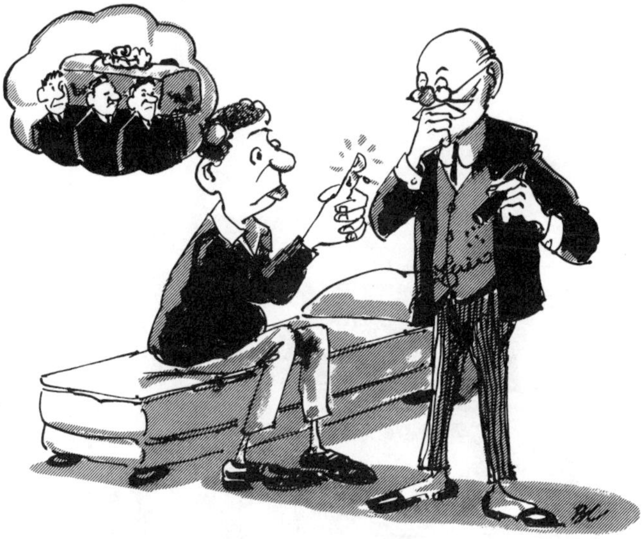

Hypochondriasis

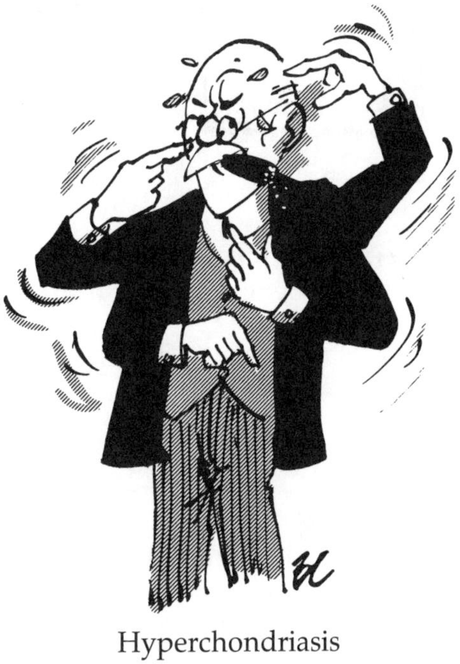

Hyperchondriasis

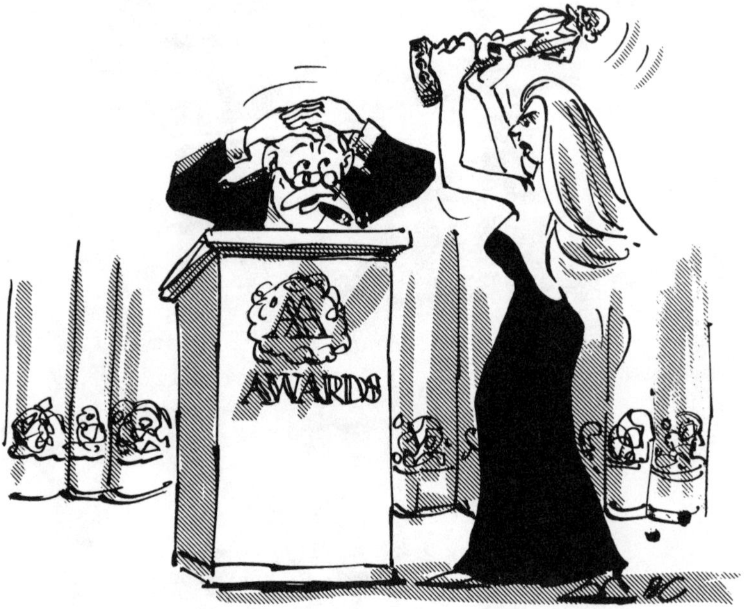

"And the award for biggest hissy fit due to a loss in another category goes to. . ."

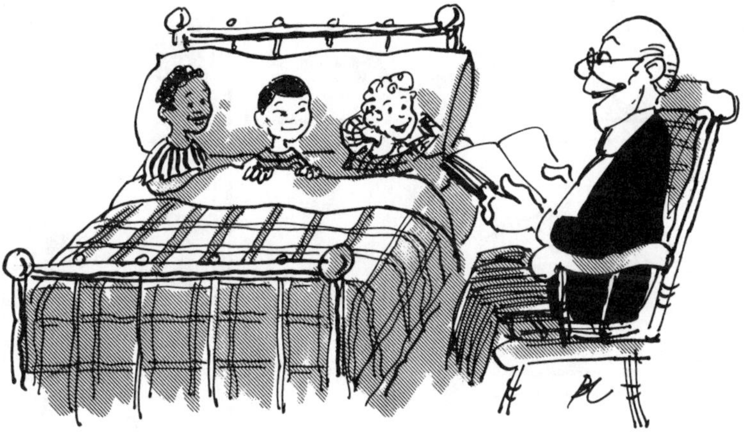

"I've been feeling down for most of the day,
nearly every day now for almost two weeks,"
said Dick to Jane.
"What do you think the problem might be?"

Paranopoly

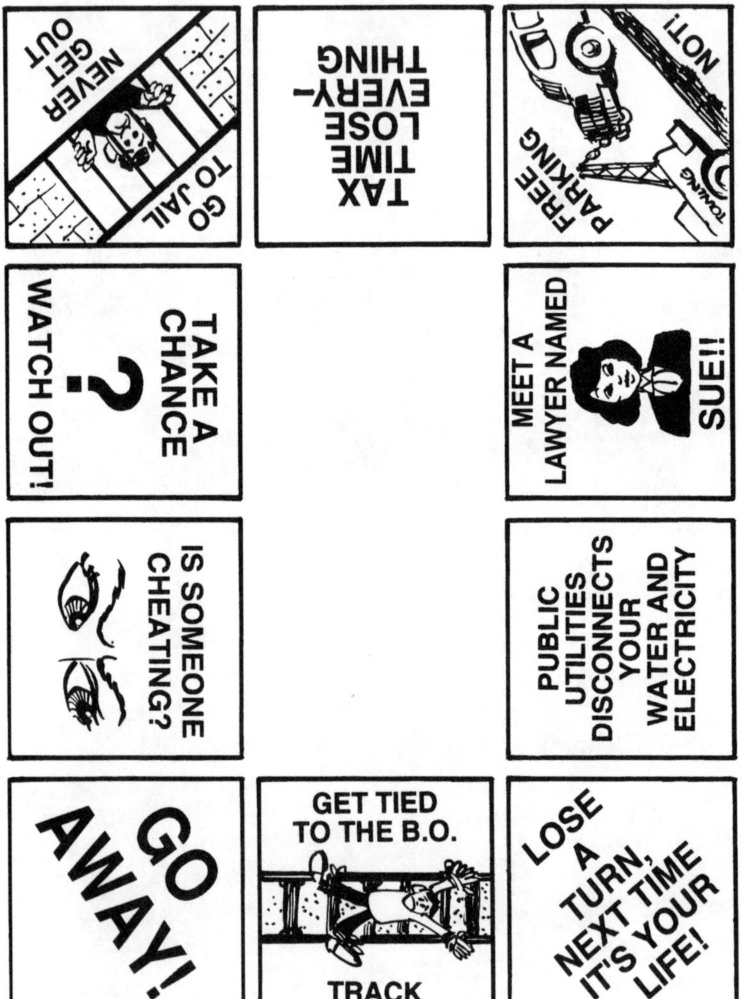
GO TO JAIL
NEVER GET OUT
TAX TIME LOSE EVERY-THING
FREE PARKING
NOT!
TOWING
TAKE A CHANCE
?
WATCH OUT!
MEET A LAWYER NAMED
SUE!!
IS SOMEONE CHEATING?
PUBLIC UTILITIES DISCONNECTS YOUR WATER AND ELECTRICITY
GO AWAY!
GET TIED TO THE B.O.
TRACK
LOSE A TURN, NEXT TIME IT'S YOUR LIFE!

Chapter 10.
The Daily Grind

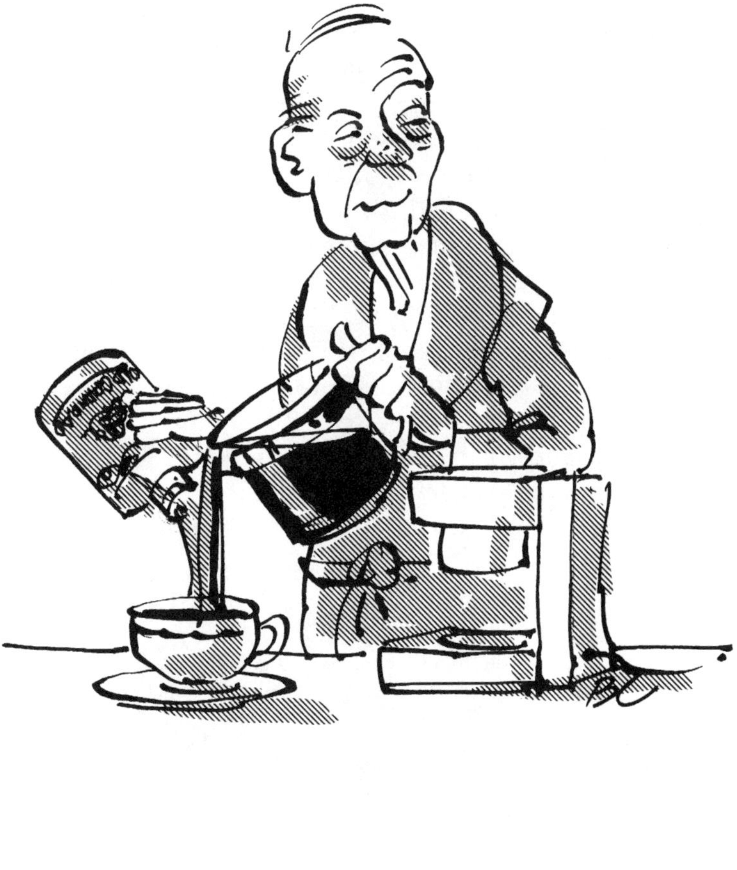

The Impact of Hissy Fits

W.E. Osmun, M.D. and C. Naugler, M.D.

And when the hissy fit was on him, I did mark how he did shake.
— *William Shakespeare,* Julius Caesar

Although hissy fits are common, there is scant information on them in the medical literature. They affect our lives daily and have been known to originate from both physician and patient. One of a number of obnoxious behaviours, hissy fits have never been studied to determine their full impact. Our search of MEDLINE using the MeSH terms "hissy" and "fit" retrieved few articles. Watson and Crick[a] in their seminal paper on the structure of DNA,[1] failed to locate a hissy fit locus, indeed they failed to mention hissy fits at all. The Human Genome Project,[b] hoping to remedy this, also failed.[2] The evolutionary advantage of hissy fits has never been fully explored, Darwin[c] feeling that birds with sticks were of greater interest than his fellow humans.[3] Freud,[d] plunging into mankind's subconscious, found the subject of hissy fits so threatening that he repressed all mention of them in his writings, preferring to deal only in mythical allegories.[e4] Although it can be conjectured that a hissy fit would be an excellent source of clean power, the scientific community prefers to concentrate on cold fusion.

[a] We don't know what the fuss is about these 2 guys. The way everyone talks about them, you'd think they had invented the Slinky or something.
[b] We have no idea what the Human Genome Project is.
[c] Also the name of an Australian city.
[d] Try telling us this guy wasn't a little obsessed with the naughty bits.
[e] Like that whole Oedipus thing, sick or what?
[f] This guy's so famous they've named whole, entire fields after him. We'd rather they name a library after us.

Banting and Best[5] neglected to mention that hypoglycemia could well be the cause of many hissy fits. Pasteur[f] was unable to identify an infectious agent resulting in hissy fits, which is all for the best because Fleming[6] found that hissy fits were not controllable with penicillin. There is a paucity of literature on hissy fits. We hope that our study will begin to open the window on this behaviour and one day lead to a cure.

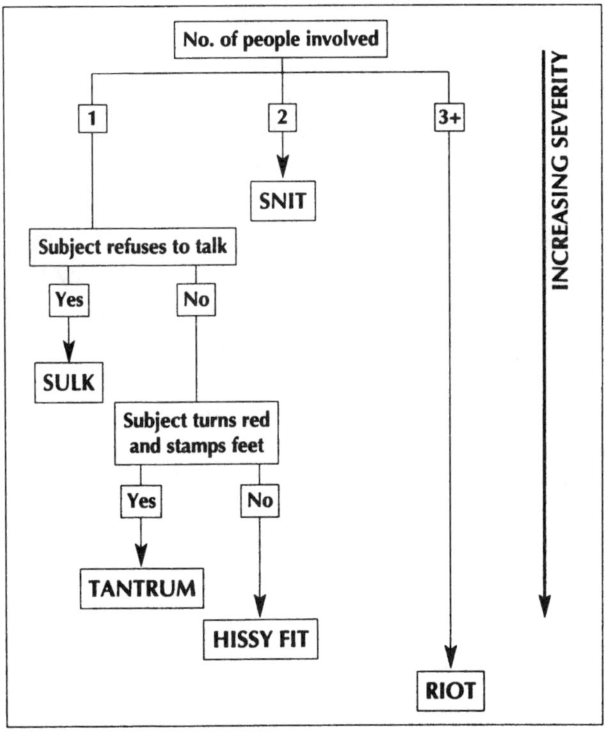

Fig. 1: Naugler–Osmun Hissy Fit Identification System

Methods

Our study was conducted over 12 months at the Happy Valley Clinic, a multidisciplinary teaching clinic of a university in Ontario. This clinic serves a mixed population of aging

Lotharios, Latin American dancers and seedy, professorial types. It enjoys 20 000 visits a year, mainly for strained groin muscles. Research assistants were trained to identify hissy fits using the Naugler–Osmun Hissy Fit Identification System ($9.95; patent pending) (Fig. 1). Initially two research assistants were stationed strategically at the clinic 24 hours a day, but it became apparent to the researchers that, because there were no patients or staff on duty between 5 pm and 8 am, there were few hissy fits to be observed then. Therefore, we limited our study to working hours only.

Results

We soon discovered that hissy fits were common at our clinic. There was a definite seasonal variation, with fits being much more common in November and December, except for a peak in July that coincided with air conditioner malfunction. Failure to prescribe antibiotics for upper respiratory infections and to support workers compensation claims for hot tubs for pulled groin muscles were the most frequent causes of hissy fits that originated from patients. Physician-generated hissy fits were usually a result of patients calling at 4:59 pm asking to be seen immediately for a groin pull they had had for several days. A group hissy fit (also known as a riot) was observed when the residents were refused permission to take a day off en masse to attend a CME event (a Céline Dion concert).[g] The damage incurred resulted in the clinic being closed for repairs for a week in September. One staff person threw a hissy fit when his residents failed to acknowledge his birthday.[h] Perpetrators of hissy fits were interviewed by the research assistants. All agreed that the fit resulted in feelings of relief.

[g] They got tickets from a drug company. We try to discourage this sort of behaviour, but what can you do?

[h] That was me (W.E.O.), and I feel the fit was totally justified. I also feel it wasn't really a hissy fit, more of a snit.

[i] What a bunch of no-hoper, do-gooder losers, they should all go out and get a life and stop sticking their nose in other people's groundbreaking clinical research.

Comments ranged from "He had it coming, the #%@&*%$#!" to "Get out of my face, you @#$%&^% or I'll show you a real hissy fit."

The victims of hissy fits uniformly felt that they had been unreasonably treated. Comments ranged from a shrug to "Do you have the number of the University Harassment Officer?"

Witnesses were interviewed as to the emotional impact. Comments ranged from "What's a hissy fit?" to "She should grow up." None said that having witnessed a hissy fit interfered with their emotional or physical health.

Interpretation

It is apparent that a number of obnoxious behaviours are prevalent in a community clinic. Care must be taken not to allow hissy fits to escalate into riots. Riots often lead to destruction of the physical plant, which may interrupt the provision of important medical care to the patient population. The victims of hissy fits interviewed found them quite distressing. It may help to have sublingual Ativan on hand for the victims. Sublingual Ativan may also be useful if administered early to a hissy fitter, to attenuate the attack. Other methods of hissy fit prophylaxis need to be developed.

Unfortunately, our proposal for a double-blind, randomized controlled trial of the effect of electric cattle prods on hissy fit behaviour was rejected by the University Ethics Board.[i]

Conclusion

Hissy fits are an important expression of angst in our society. Nevertheless, victims find them quite distressing. Every effort should be made to counsel hissy fitters on how best to control their behaviour and channel their aggressions into more socially acceptable behaviours.

References

1. Watson, Dr., and Crick, Jiminy. The discovery of twisty things. *The Naturist* 1960; 7:10-5.

2. Kimbrell A. *The human body shop*. New York: HarperSanFrancisco; 1993.

3. Darwin, Charles. *The origin of species*. Published so long ago, who cares where, when and by whom?

4. Freud, Sigmund (Siggy to his friends). This guy wrote so many books, we couldn't decide which one to cite. So if you're really interested, why don't you show a little initiative and go look him up in the library. We're tired of doing all the work for you.

5. Banting and Best. Like, these guys are so famous down 'round here that we don't figure we should have to tell you more. We think they invented the Slinky.

6. Fleming, forgot his first name. He's the guy that went a bit mouldy, and he wasn't even dead yet!

Reprinted with permission of the Canadian Medical Association Journal.
This article was originally published in:
CMAJ • DEC. 15, 1998; 159 (12) 1457 — 1459

An Improved Psychiatric Consult Form

Robert S. Hoffman, M.D.

Over the years there have been a number of attempts to devise a standardized form for psychiatric consultations. Regrettably, these forms bear little, if any, relationship to the questions most frequently posed by referring sources. Our initial study involved polling a group (n=6½) of non-psychiatric physicians to determine the information they desired from psychiatric consultations. Notably, all respondents returned blank pieces of paper. In a second study, these physicians were re-contacted and offered $65 to participate. This time they all responded and overwhelmingly indicated that the information in a typical consultation note was obtuse, boring, and useless. One respondent indicated a preference for illegible write-ups over legible ones. Over 80% of the sample rarely requested psychiatric consultation. When asked if anything could be done to improve the quality of referral notes, the majority indicated that shortening the length of reports would be the most important change. The results of their specific suggestions are incorporated into the form presented on the next two pages.

References

Jung, C.G: *Use of the Mandala in Consultation-Liaison Psychiatry*
Swiss J. of Gen. Hosp. Mythology, Vol. 16 (4), 1918, p. 13-133

Stein, G: *A Form is a Form is a Form*
Archives of Verbigeration, Vol. 2 (2), 1922, p. 2-22

Grover, E: *The Therapeutic Effect of Inexact Consultation: A Contribution to the Theory of Obfuscation*
Int. J. of Psychoankylosis, Vol. (12), 1931, p. 397-411

Psychiatric Consultation Form

In order to maintain confidentiality, do not indicate the patient's name anywhere on this form

Reason for consultation (to be filled in by referring source):

1. Talk with the patient until he/she is calm.
2. Transfer to the psychiatry inpatient unit **stat**.
3. Sedate until obtunded.
4. Evaluate the patient and start a medication.
5. Treat as required, but do not involve the referring source in any way.

Consultant's Report

History of Present Illness:

1. Has troubles
2. Does not have troubles

Mental Status Examination:

General Behavior	__ insufferable
	__ intolerable
	__ incontinent
Mood	__ up
	__ down
	__ neither up nor down
Thought Process	__ tight
	__ loose
	__ thought processor on *frappé*
Thought Content	__ focused
	__ out of focus
	__ out of film

Judgment	__	agrees with consultant
	__	disagrees with consultant
	__	vacillates like a politician
Cognition	__	understands Shakespeare
	__	understands sitcoms
	__	understands commercials

Diagnostic Impression:

1. Happy		
2. Sad	__	loused-up life situation
	__	loused-up brain chemistry
3. Mad		
4. Bad	__	hysterical
	__	malingering
	__	compensation neurosis
	__	drug-seeking behavior
	__	without health insurance

Certainty of Diagnosis:

__ snowball's chance
__ lottery-ticket odds

Psychodynamic Understanding:

__ have one
__ don't have one

Recommendations:

1. Transfer to psychiatry.
2. Start an:

   __ anti-psychotic
   __ anti-neurotic
   __ anti-biotic
   __ anti-spasmodic
   __ attitude suppressant

This is a modified version of an article originally printed in the *Journal of Therapeutic Humor*, Summer 1981, Vol. 1(2). Reprinted with permission.

Rationale for Requesting Consults

David J. Robinson, M.D.

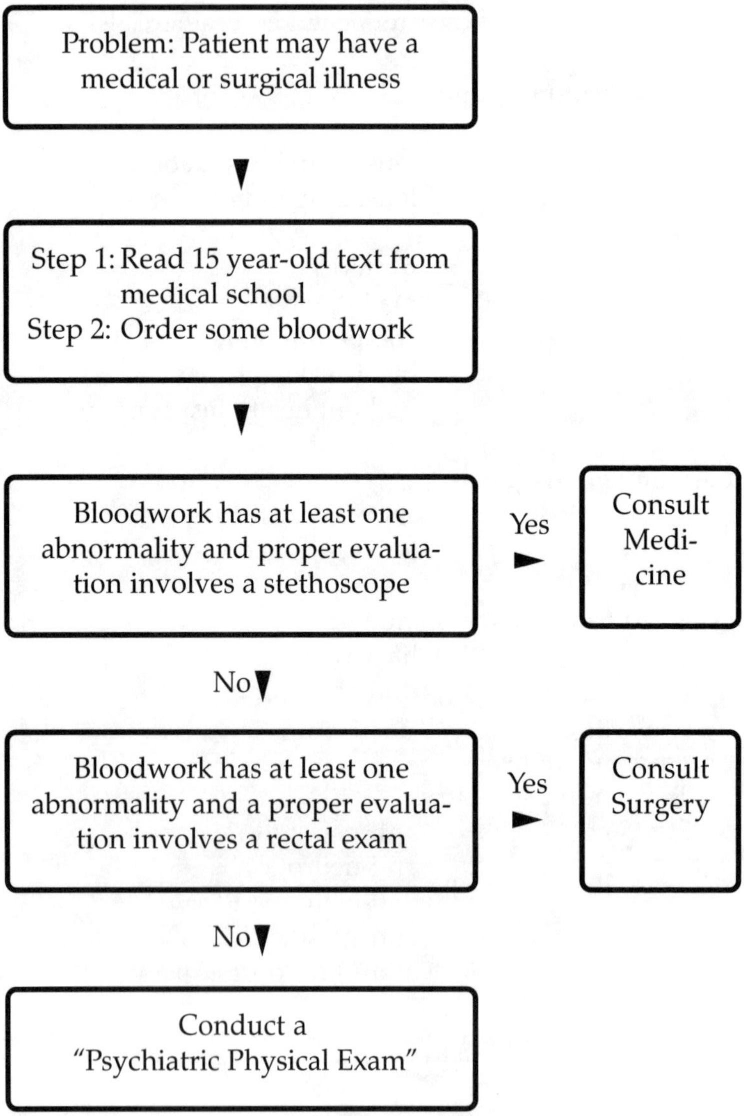
Problem: Patient may have a medical or surgical illness
Step 1: Read 15 year-old text from medical school
Step 2: Order some bloodwork
Bloodwork has at least one abnormality and proper evaluation involves a stethoscope
Yes
Consult Medicine
No
Bloodwork has at least one abnormality and a proper evaluation involves a rectal exam
Yes
Consult Surgery
No
Conduct a "Psychiatric Physical Exam"

The Psychiatric Physical Exam

David J. Robinson, M.D.

Cranial Nerve Assessment

Maneuver/Activity	Tests
Ask patient to visually track a flashlight waved in front of eyes	Cranial nerves (CN) 2 (sees light) 3, 4, 6 (follows light)
Impale flashlight in patient's eye	CN 5 (corneal reflex)
Stand behind patient and break wind	CN 1 (smell) 7 (winces), 8 (sound), 11 (turns head)
Ask patient to protrude tongue	CN 12 (tongue control)
Gag patient with tongue depressor	CN 9 and 10 (gag control)

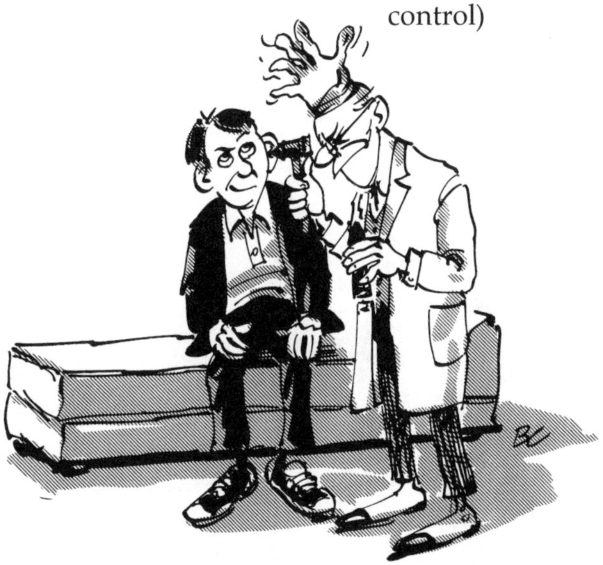

Cardiovascular System

(Two of three required)
Can the patient. . .

❑ Run out of the ER fast enough to elude the police?

❑ Go to the drugstore to get the machine to take his or her pulse and blood pressure?

❑ Afford an EKG?

Respiratory System

(Two of three required)
Can the patient. . .

❑ Show you nicotine stains from cigarettes?

❑ Yell at his or her spouse?

❑ Launch a spitball?

Fine Motor Control

(Two of three required)
Can the patient. . .

❑ Light a cigarette?

❑ Find Canadian pennies in a handful of coins?

❑ Use a vending machine?

Gross Motor Control

(One of two required)
Can the patient. . .

❑ Go to the store to buy cigarettes

❑ Find the piece missing from the inpatient unit puzzle

Gastrointestinal System

(Two of three required)
Can the patient. . .

- ❑ Digest fast-food?
- ❑ Break wind to retaliate for your cranial nerve exam?
- ❑ Belch the first few bars of a popular song?

Genitourinary System

(Two of three required)
Can the patient. . .

- ❑ Spell gynecologist or urologist?
- ❑ Wait until the end of the interview before answering nature's call?
- ❑ Handle light, regular, and heavy beer?

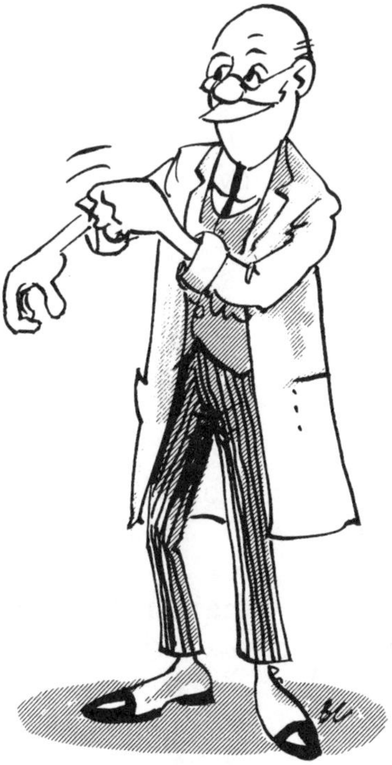

"Teach medical students how to peform a rectal exam and they will learn.

Force them to perform rectal exams and they become psychiatrists"

Dr. I. Finger
Early 20st Century
Physician
London, England

CyberTherapy Update:

Contamination Risks via Computer Virus

Jay Ryser, M.Ed. & James Buckingham, M.D.
Lakewood, Colorado & Nagochdoches, Texas

As the Internet and the World Wide Web become more ubiquitous, "CyberTherapy" is becoming a more common, and for some, a more accessible source of treatment for emotional difficulties. Licensure and standards for treatment struggle to keep pace with technology in this burgeoning field. An often neglected component is not how technology affects treatment, but how treatment affects technology. CyberTherapist and CyberClient alike, are with alarming frequency, reporting new strains of computer viruses unique to the CyberTherapy field. An cataloging of the more widespread and malignant viruses is included in this article.

Common CyberTreatment Viruses (Virii?)

- **Fugue State Virus**: causes a treatment file to disappear, which then resurfaces on an entirely different drive under a different name several days later

- **Anorexic Virus**: attacks and eliminates the File Allocation Table (FAT)

- **Bulimic Virus**: consumes the largest files on the hard disk then purges them into the desktop Trash Can/Recycle Bin

- **Dissociative Identity Virus**: fragments the hard drive into multiple smaller drives that won't recognize each other and refuse to share data

- **Paranoid Virus**: asks for your password before it allows you to open each file and informs you repeatedly that the World Wide Web is a United Nations conspiracy

- **Borderline — Type 1 Virus**: splits the hard disc into two separate drives

- **Borderline — Type 2 Virus**: deletes the video drivers and forces the screen to display in only black and white

- **Borderline — Type 3 (a.k.a. Lorena Bobbit) Virus**: turns your hard disk into a 3½″ floppy

- **Borderline — Type 4 Virus**: uses the modem to call Cyber-Therapist at 3 A.M. with threats to slash wrist rests

- **Sociopathic Virus**: uses your *.BAT* files to trash all the other files, then e-mails your credit information to inmates at the Texas Department of Criminal Justice

- **Narcissistic Virus**: exaggerates the value of computer components (i.e. larger hard drive, more memory, faster CPU speed, etc. than the system actually has)

- **Alzheimer's Virus**: computer forgets where it has stored files, then displays the wrong date and time, forgets your e-mail address and then can't find your home page

- **Narcoleptic Virus**: activates the screen saver at random intervals

- **Phobic Virus**: uses a *.WAV* file to scream whenever the mouse is used

- **Tourette's Virus**: causes the screen to blink many times each minute, then uses .WAV files to blurt out random obscenities

- **Passive-Aggressive Virus**: reboots the computer when you try to save a file, reports *.DLL* and *.EXE* files are missing when they are plainly in the system, reports your passwords are no longer valid and finally deletes your e-mail before you have a chance to read it

- **Hypochondriasis Virus**: computer constantly alerts you it has a virus despite antivirus software's failure to locate any virus, repeatedly requests you call technical support for advice, and wants you to run diagnostic software at the start of every application

- **Obsessive-Compulsive Virus**: refuses to delete files because you might need them again someday, optimizes hard disk so frequently that you can't do any work, won't let you print a file until it has run a spell check and grammar check several times, constantly checks disk integrity, continually reminds you to back up your data, and refuses to read data from other sources for fear of contamination

- **Panic Virus**: reports continuous *Fatal Disk Error* messages despite normal hard disk functioning

- **Agoraphobia Virus**: same as above, but infects laptop and notebook computer exclusively so that they refuse to boot up anywhere other than at home

- **Depression Virus**: slows CPU speed by 50%, system is reluctant to boot up, has diminished memory, decreased energy consumption, blames itself for every *General Protection Fault*, reminds you how obsolete it is, and discourages technical support because, "It just won't help."

- **PMS Virus**: mouse pad disappears every month

- **Histrionic Virus**: changes default fonts to the large, bold, dramatic fonts and then changes the system wallpaper

- **Schizophrenic Virus**: reports *command.com* hallucinations, fears Bill Gates is the Anti-Christ, *Dial-Up Networking* won't connect

- **Exhibitionist Virus**: exposes hard drive, brags about size

- **Cult Virus**: requires extensive deprogramming

- **Occult Virus**: writes "666" each time a key is pressed

- **False Memory Virus**: shows list of websites in your cache that you've never actually visited

Commonly Found Viruses Specific to CyberTherapists' Computers

- **Freud Virus**: the computer becomes obsessed with its own motherboard

- **Ellis Virus**: deletes the words *should, ought, must, awful, horrible,* and *catastrophic* from word processor dictionaries, grammar checker constantly requests you to reword the paragraph to e-prime, then claims all other virii are ineffective

- **Rogers Virus**: re-displays every sentence you type and includes an occasional "um-hmm"

- **ECT Virus**: instructs you to decrease system memory without first unplugging the computer

- **Aversive Virus**: administers harmless but painful shock through the keyboard in the event of a misspellink (ow!)

Acronymilalia

Jane P. Sheldon, Ph.D.
University of Michigan-Dearborn

Recently, in the therapy setting, a new disordered behavior has been identified in which the client's speech is filled with shortened phrases and codes to the point where no sentence can be uttered without one. This condition, known as **acronymilalia**, can greatly impair the client's ability to communicate. It may also be associated with obsessive-compulsive disorder. The following excerpt from a therapy session is illustrative of the condition:

Therapist: "Last time you were here you said you weren't feeling well. How are you doing this week?"

Client: "PU. A trip to my MD earlier this week showed that my BP is above normal. HDL levels are fine, though. And, no HIV (AKA AIDS). EKG results TBA. Their ETA is Tuesday. I was PO'd that my SOB doctor wouldn't show me some TLC and do an EEG, cuz my brain still feels wired. Don't worry, I'm not ready for RIP or anything, but I'm getting close to going AWOL, if you know what I mean. TGIF. I need some R & R."

Acronymilalia may involve a biological component, yet it is evident that certain environmental contingencies play a role in its etiology. Just as with substance use, individuals with the tendency towards this condition are highly influenced by being with others who have this disorder. FYI: Symptoms can appear PDQ, even when a few minutes before everything was OK. Because this abnormal behavior is not included in the DSM, it is imperative that the APA recognizes the disorder ASAP.

Chapter 11. Top 5 Lists

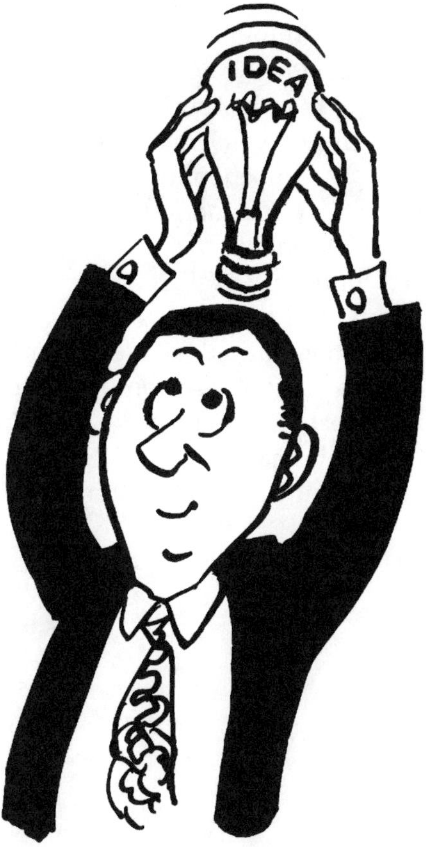

The Top 13 Little Known Phobias

13. "Hey, this is a nude beach! I ain't getting in that cold water!" — Shrinkaphobia
12. "Get that #$%#-ing vodka bottle away from me!!" — Carmenelectraphobia
11. "He's coming straight for us — with his left turn signal on!" — Oldfartophobia
10. "You have to push 'Start' to turn the damn computer off?!" — Windophobia
9. "I won't go to your frat house to eat gyros and watch a tape of the Israel Philharmonic Orchestra on your old Sony VCR!" — ThetaFetaMehtaBetaphobia
8. "Tonight on Paramount: 'Come quickly Gabrielle! We must s" <click!> — Xenaphobia
7. "NO!! Don't call the plumber!!!" — Buttcrackophobia
6. "No, I don't want to watch 'Friends'. That blonde chick freaks me out." — Phoebephobia
5. "Uhm, Doctor, why are you putting on that rubber glove?" — Probeophobia
4. "You're busy Saturday? Well, how about next weekend then?" — Rentanotherpornophobia
3. "It's NOT my imagination! Senator Helms is looking at me *that* way again!" — Homophobophobia
2. "Wait! If we impeach him, then the new President will be..."— aGoreophobia
1. "Honey, I bought a Corvette!" — Smallpeniphobia

The Top 13 Signs Your Sexual Fetish Is Out of Control

13. It's difficult to find a woman willing to dress up as Strom Thurmond.
12. You'd think Tara Lipinski would at least say "Thank you" for the 562-page collage and poems. But noooooooooo...
11. Your fixation with weird gadgets has led you to propose to Carrot Top.
10. Your local TV news has warned women more than once about wearing open-toed shoes after eating garlic.
9. Human Resources has to inform you that "business casual" does not include latex.
8. Thanks to you, a whole generation of Great Pandas have forgotten how to reproduce without Pink Floyd, peanut butter and "Professor Leather."
7. You get visibly aroused every time you hear Skitch Henderson's version of "It's a Grand Old Flag."
6. You're being treated for your foot fetish by Dr. Scholl himself.
5. The restraining order from PETA was inevitable, but now you've been banned from KFC in 32 states.
4. The other astronauts all declined your offer to join the "600 Mile High Club."
3. Eighty-seven garden gnomes on the lawn — but oh, baby, does your body hunger for more.
2. The highlight of your ski vacation was putting the snow chains on your tires.
1. Your wife takes your little game too far and gets elected Senator from New York.

The Top 14 Least-Known Psychological Afflictions

14. Elevitis: The compulsive need to press already-lit elevator buttons.
13. Shoshanism: Persistent, pathological fascination with persons of no discernible accomplishment beyond their former association with celebrities. (See also Katotonia, Monicanucleosis)
12. Schlitzophrenia: The inexplicable desire to consume cheap domestic beer.
11. Munchies-Syndrome-By-Proxy: A craving for salty snack foods, often triggered by the pot smoking of others.
10. Fallonian Denial: Recurring belief that maybe, just maybe, this week's "Saturday Night Live" won't suck.
9. Bull-imia: Self-destructive cycle of bingeing on blue chips, then purging stocks at market close.
8. Chadophobia: Irrational fear you might suddenly punch a passing Floridian.
7. Dietrrhea: The inability to be on a weight-loss program without talking about it to everyone in the tri-state area.
6. Dubyalusions of Grandeur: Mistaken belief that you actually won the election.
5. Adolescinemaphilia: Uncontrollable urge to see a Freddie Prinze, Jr. movie.
4. Probst-Traumatic Stress Disorder: Fear of being voted out of the tribe.
3. White's Syndrome: The inability to compile a list that conforms with pre-determined numerical criteria.
2. Bipolarbear Disorder: Desire to have sex with large arctic carnivores of either gender.
1. Barcolepsy: The inability to remain awake for longer than 30 seconds after sitting in the recliner in front of the TV.

Reprinted with permission courtesy of TopFive.com

The Top 13 Signs Your Radio "Psychiatrist" Has Posed Nude

13. Her station's new slogan: "More Talk, Less Clothes!"
12. Her cure for people's fear of public speaking no longer requires any imagination.
11. Photo on her driver's license taken by Bob Guccione.
10. Pompous elitist attitude a direct result of the camera making her look 10 lbs. heavier.
9. Her standard on-air greeting: "This is Dr. Laura, and I'm naked."
8. Now rails on the importance of keeping all nine commandments.
7. "Hello, this is Dr. Laura Schlessinger. I am my children's hypocritical, adulterous, boney-assed mom."
6. Her nickname in the studio? "Dr. Bareassinger."
5. That twirling tassel she uses for hypnosis.
4. She ends your session with, "You know, Hef has a couch just like this."
3. Insists on being called "Dr. November 1978"
2. Keeps asking, "Does this notepad make my ass look big?"
1. Screams "How 'bout them Yankees?!" every time a caller mentions nude photos.

The Top 10 Freudian Pick-Up Lines

10. Your superego may be saying "no" but your id is giving me a tongue bath.

9. Wanna come back to my place and do something you'll repress later?

8. Did I tell you I'm a Certified Pubic Accountant?

7. Y'know, a few minutes of probing on my couch and you'd be a completely different woman.

6. You remind me of my mother when she was Jung.

5. I'll envy yours if you envy mine

4. I believe in putting the "psycho" back in "psychoanalysis."

3. Can I buy you a shrink?

2. . . . Ooops! I meant *Horatio*! My name is *Horatio*.

1. . . . unt ven I schnap my fingers, you vill put your clothes back on unt remember none of zees. . .

Reprinted with permission courtesy of TopFive.com

The Top 8 Signs Your Inner Child is Unhappy

8. Hasn't touched your inner train set for days.

7. You attempt to overdose on a lethal combination of J & B and M & M's.

6. When you try to hug him, he pulls away and calls you a "pathetic codependent loser."

5. Has been sulking since you refused to buy that Power Ranger doll.

4. Keeps getting thrown out of bars for ordering Lucky Charms and milk.

3. Primal scream portion of "Bert & Ernie's Anger Management Workshop" has kept you up three nights in a row.

2. Sudden urge to knock your morning cappuccino and bagel on the floor.

1. You keep your therapist at bay with a Lego Uzi until the Gummi Bear ransom has arrived.

The Top 10 Rejected Self-Help Books

10. Listening to Pez
9. Toilet Training Your Inner Child
8. The One-Step-Forward, Two-Steps-Backward Program for the Chronically Indecisive
7. Losing Weight Slowly by Eating Less and Exercising
6. Drink Yourself Sober
5. Old & Barren: Embracing Your Inner Spinster
4. "Thank Vishnu for Neurotic White Folks" by Deepak Chopra
3. "I'm OK, You're Going to Hell" by Ralph Reed
2. The One Minute Lover
1. Heart to Huh? Monosyllabic Communication with the Man in Your Life

The Top 8 Signs You Need to Find A New Support Group

8. The name: *Promise Breakers*
7. *Parents Without Partners* survey — 18 members, 18 beards.
6. Four months and the *Nymphomania Group* still hasn't recruited a female member.
5. Instead of Mars and Venus, leader suggests you get in touch with Uranus.
4. You're the host for the upcoming pool party for your *Incontinent Beer Drinkers Support Group*.
3. Their idea of 12 Steps consists of two six-packs.
2. Only an hour into the meeting and the keg's already dry.
1. Group: *Anorexics Anonymous*. You: Big chubby guy with an affinity for cheesecake.

The Top 10 Signs the Santa at the Mall is Nuts

10. Shaves head and beard, insists on being called "Santa Kurtz."

9. The twinkle in his eye and the twitch of his nose are due to a lack of psychotropic medication.

8. Has a complimentary tray of "Tundra Oysters" ready for the toddlers.

7. Actually enjoys it when small children urinate on his lap.

6. Answers every child's toy request with, "Dream on, pee wee."

5. Despite substantial evidence to the contrary, claims to never have worn white gloves or shiny black boots.

4. Tells kids about the comparative kill ratio of the AK-47 over the Nerf Dart Gun.

3. When a child wets his lap, he returns the favor.

2. Instead of a candy cane, he gives each kid a pack of Marlboros and piece of homemade venison pie.

1. While it's admittedly a nifty trick, blowing smoke rings out of his tracheotomy hole is scaring the hell out of the kiddies.

The Top 10 Indications Your Family May be Dysfunctional

10. Your vacations are planned through AA instead of AAA.

9. Your mother and preteen sister always fight over the last beer.

8. In the middle of a family reunion, the FBI cuts power to the ranch.

7. You have to buy separate Mother's Day cards for each of Mom's personalities.

6. Family discussions usually begin with, "Put the gun down."

5. Thanksgiving Dinner consists of Wild Turkey instead of roast turkey.

4. You finally get your work published in a major newspaper and your brother rats you out to the Feds.

3. The bikers next door are always complaining about the noise.

2. Your new little sister is named after a famous serial killer.

1. Your brother is writing a nostalgic screenplay entitled, "A Menendez Family Christmas."

Reprinted with permission courtesy of TopFive.com

The Top 9 Signs Your Kid Will Grow Up to be a Criminal

9. Uses lemonade stand as a front to sell your jewelry.

8. Always banging cup against crib bars.

7. Wears her mom's nylons — over her head.

6. Her "Weebles" keep knocking over the Playskool bank.

5. "Squealers" end up floating face down in Mr. Turtle pool.

4. Hasn't taken his first step yet, but has already, "taken the fifth."

3. Stubbornly refuses to put the cat back together.

2. Shaves her Ken's doll hair into a Mohawk to make a homemade Travis Bickle action figure.

1. Always willing to trade hotels on Boardwalk for "Get Out of Jail Free cards" in Monopoly.

The Top 9 Signs Your Cat Has a Personality Disorder

9. Teeth and claw marks over your now-empty bottle of Prozac.

8. No longer licks paws clean, but washes them in the sink again and again and again.

7. Continually scratches at the door to get in . . the OVEN door.

6. Rides in your car with its head out the window.

5. Doesn't get Garfield, but laughs like hell at Marmaduke.

4. Your stereo is missing and in the corner you find a pawn ticket and 2 kilos of catnip.

3. Spends all day in litterbox separating the green chlorophyll granules from the plain white ones.

2. Makes a shrine to Andrew Lloyd Webber out of empty "9 Lives" cans.

1. Makes an attempt on "First Cat" Sock's life in a pathetic attempt to impress Jodie Foster.

The Top 8 Threats Used in Dysfunctional Families

8. "Finish your lima beans or you're not getting any heroin for dessert!"

7. "If this plexiglass wasn't between us, I'd wash your mouth out with soap, young man."

6. "Eat you Brussels sprouts or Mommy won't love you anymore."

5. "Lyle, Eric — either behave or go back to your suites."

4. "Don't make me put you back in the womb."

3. "As long as you live in this house, you're going to wear that dress, young man!"

2. "You just wait until your father gets paroled."

1. "Stop crying Lourdes, or Uncle Dennis will kick you in the groin."

Reprinted with permission courtesy of TopFive.com

The Top 11 Signs Your Doctor Doesn't Like You

11. Tells you smoking is no more harmful than drinking.

10. Anesthesia? A shot of Wild Turkey and a good swift karate chop.

9. Insists the entire exam can be done via email.

8. For cirrhosis, recommends "a hair of the hound that bit you."

7. Has you lie down and instructs the nurse to "fetch a big ol' IV of pork drippin's."

6. Keeps your tongue depressor in his loafers.

5. After weighing you, gets on the office intercom and announces, "two-hundred and forty-five pounds, we have a winnah!"

4. After the physical? Never writes, never calls.

3. Bill reads, "Balance due immediately, or we'll tell everyone about the herpes."

2. While under anesthesia, tattoos "Danger: Gas" on your butt.

1. Gives, rather than takes urine samples.

The Top 10 Signs You Suffer From Road Rage (I)

10. Driver's license exam question; "When passing on the right, always __________? Your answer; Shoot to kill.

9. State Farm refuses to insure a personal vehicle with gun turrets.

8. You've packed enough guns and ammo to make a Tarantino film yet you're only going to the store to buy milk.

7. Your blood pressure is higher than Ditka's.

6. Someone cuts you off and the next thing you know, two members of your carpool get killed in the crossfire.

5. You've developed carpal tunnel syndrome in your middle finger.

4. A) Teeth marks on the steering wheel all the way down to the 5 and 7 o'clock positions; B) You're not Christian Slater, Mike Tyson or Marv Albert

3. Left arm bigger than Popeye's from giving the finger and aiming the Uzi.

2. Lazy chopper pilot for Fox TV's "Real Crashes" simply waits in the vacant lot next to your garage.

1. You can't resist firing off a few practice shots whenever you pass a target store.

Reprinted with permission courtesy of TopFive.com

The Top 7 Signs You Suffer From Road Rage (II)

7. For lack of a more effective weapon, you find yourself threatening other drivers with the cigarette lighter.

6. Local Crips now have a hand signal for "Get Off the Road, That Psycho's Coming!"

5. Your need to wring Dr. Laura Schlessinger's neck is just a bit more urgent than usual.

4. You swear more before you get to work than most gangsta rappers do all day.

3. The car is a year old; you're already on your fifth horn.

2. You threaten to run over the person in front of you, even though you're in line for communion.

1. On your license, under restrictions, it says "valium required."

Reprinted with permission courtesy of TopFive.com

Chapter 12.
Unclassifieds

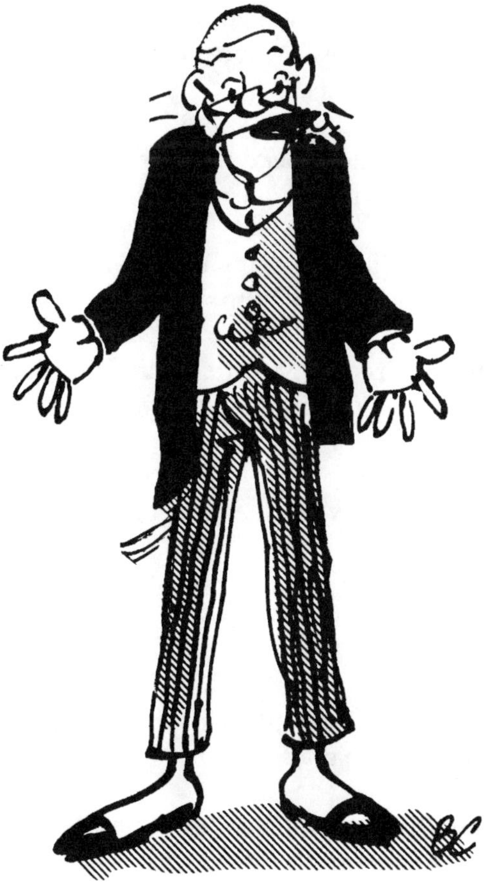

Borderlines

(Sung to the song "Borderline" by Madonna)

Lauren D. LaPorta, M.D.
Maywood, New Jersey

Doctor, can't you help me please, my life's a total mess —
I'm an addicted mutilator under lots of stress.
My boyfriend stole my car, I wanna be a star,
My mother was a selfish witch.
Need a pill for my disease, give me more of these,
Already taken five or six.

Just try to understand, I need that Ativan,
'Cause the Prozac's failing me.

Borderlines, feels like I'm going to lose my mind,
Don't know what I'm gonna to do with all of these
borderlines.
Borderlines, they're always threatening suicide,
Don't know what I'm gonna to do with all of these
borderlines.

Doctor, my moods always keep on going up and down.
In the morning, I'll be smiling, nighttime sees me with a
frown,
If my boyfriend leaves, I'll die —
I'll kill him if he tries.
I cut my wrists again last night,
Took a hundred sleeping pills, didn't pay my bills,
There seems to be no end in sight.

Just write another script, I need to be equipped,
If I go off the deep end.

Repeat chorus

Keep calling me, keep hounding me, they're driving *me* nuts,
Don't know what I'm gonna do with all of these borderlines.

I Dreamt Freud Kibbitzed With Santa Claus

(Sung to the tune of "I Saw Mommy Kissing Santa Claus")

Lauren D. LaPorta, M.D.
Maywood, New Jersey

I dreamt Freud kibbitzed with Santa Claus
Underneath the mistletoe last night.
It sure gave me the creeps,
And when I fell back to sleep,
I dreamt that they were talking 'bout the secrets that I keep.

Then I dreamt Freud was telling Santa Claus,
All the naughty things I do in spite.
Now there's coal under my tree,
Gosh, did I really see
Freud kibbitz with Santa Claus last night?

(repeat second verse)

Excellence by Assertion:

The Mount Hillary Institute

Mission Statement

The Institute will achieve unsurpassed quality empowerment paradigms in establishing itself as the "be all — end all" of mental health care for children, adolescents, adults, senior citizens, the disabled, the foul and ill-tempered, and the odoriferous and poorly groomed.

Our reputation will not end within our city or even country, but extend to the world and all known worlds. In keeping with this ambitious and noble quest, we have developed the following mission statement:

Psychiatry, the final frontier. Our ongoing mission is to:

- Seek out new patients and forms of third-party billing
- Encounter strange new populations and diagnose them
- To boldly go further than any institute has gone before

Vision

Our leader has visions and would like to share them:

"I see an institute where adults are not ashamed to seek appropriate treatment for their psychiatric disorders. I see a hospital where the chronic patients don't "cheek" medication. I see a hospital that encourages parents to follow through with their children's behavioral programs and contracts.

I see a hospital that encourages the chemically-dependent person to go to 90 meetings in 90 days and stick with one sponsor. You may say I'm a dreamer, but I'm not the only one."

Values

These are our basic corporate values:

- Complete all paperwork
- Stay in business
- Bring home a paycheck
- Don't kill anyone or screw them up too badly
- Don't do stupid, illegal, or unethical things
- Keep managed care humor to a minimum

Jay R. Ryser, M.Ed.
Lakewood, Colorado

The Bumper Sticker Principle . . .

Toward a Classification System of Psychological Subspecialties

Lillian Range Sitton, B. Jo Hailey, Gustave Sison, David C. Daniel, Jr., and Frankie Faulkner

- Academic psychologists do it with class.
- Administrative psychologists do it in triplicate.
- Behaviorists do it on schedule.
- Biofeedback researchers do it without raising their blood pressure.
- Child psychologists play like they're doing it.
- Cognitive therapists do it knowingly.
- Community psychologists do it in public.
- Consulting psychologists do it by the hour.
- Consumer psychologists use safeguards when they do it.
- Counseling psychologists do it with normals.
- Crisis interventionists do it on a moment's notice.
- Developmental psychologists do it in stages.
- Eclectic psychologists do it every possible way.
- Educational psychologists are constantly learning how to do it.
- Environmental psychologists do it organically and with out additives.
- EST therapists do it in hot tubs.
- Existential psychologists do it without thinking.
- Experimental psychologists do it with rats.
- Feminist psychologists do it N.O.W.
- Forensic psychologists do it beyond a reasonable doubt (and check for fingerprints before and after).
- Freudian psychologists do it unconsciously.
- General psychologists never do it privately.
- Gestalt psychologists do it with empty chairs.

- Group therapists do it collectively.
- Humanistic psychologists do it with feeling.
- Hypnotherapists do it suggestively.
- Industrial psychologists do it on company time.
- Jungian psychologists do it symbolically.
- Minority psychologists do it indiscriminantly.
- Music therapists use the rhythm method.
- Neo-Freudians begin doing it at a very Jung age.
- Paradoxical therapists do it backwards.
- Pastoral counselors do it in the missionary position (never standing up — it's too much like dancing).
- Pediatric psychologists do it with toys.
- Philosophical psychologists think therefore they do it.
- Physiological psychologists do it in the lab.
- Primal psychologists scream when they do it.
- Psychiatrists do it in their dreams.
- Psychoanalysts do it on the couch.
- Psychologists for the developmentally delayed do it slowly.
- Psychometricians do it in a standardized manner.
- Rational Emotive therapists don't know how Ellis to do it.
- Rogerian psychologists do it with empathy, genuineness, and warmth.
- Rorschach psychologists do it with human or animal movement.
- School psychologists do it at recess.
- Social psychologists do it in the field.
- Sex therapists are Masters at doing it.
- Statisticians do it significantly more often.
- Systematic desensitization therapists do it in successive approximations.
- TA psychologists get warm and fuzzy when they do it.
- Vocational counselors do it Strongly.

This article was originally printed in the *Journal of Therapeutic Humor*, Fall 1980, Vol. (1), No. 1. Reprinted with permission. For information, please contact:
Dr. M. Wikler, Associate Editor, JOTH
4713 — 17th Ave.
Brooklyn, NY
USA 11204

Personality Disorder Tic Tac Toe

Catherine Mallory, R.N., M.A.
London, Ontario

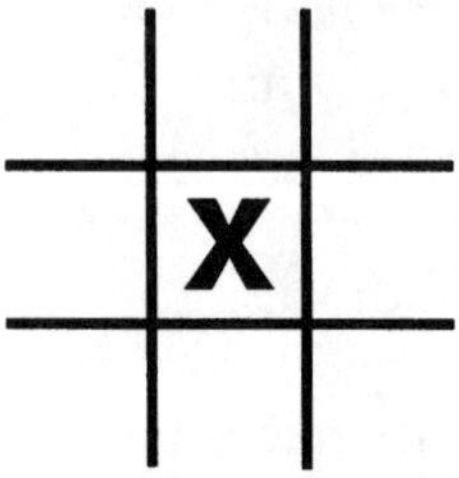

Narcissistic

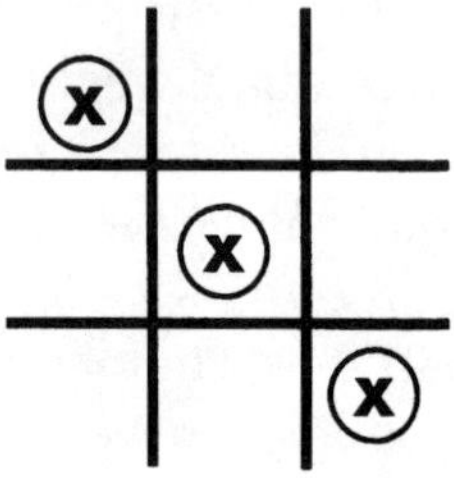

Dependent

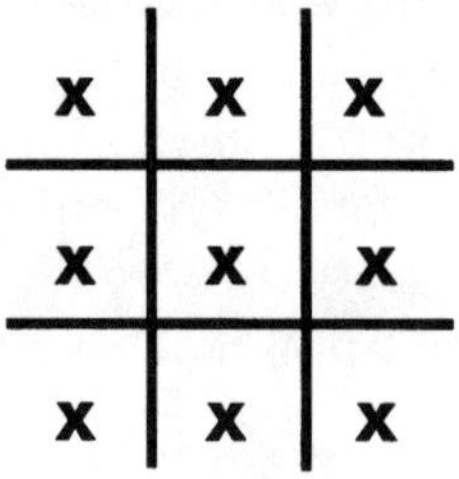

Obsessive-
Compulsive

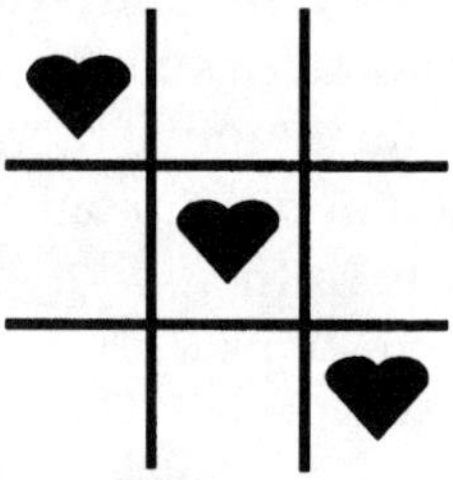

Narcissistic

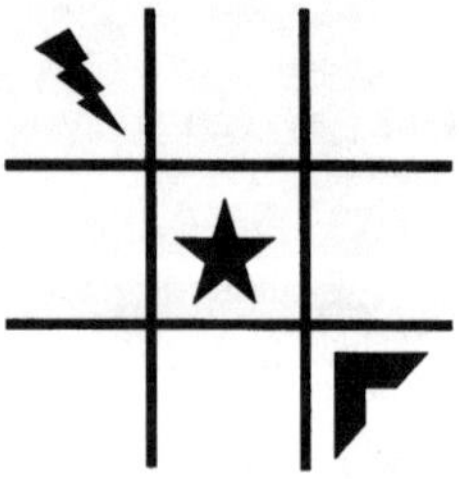

Schizotypal

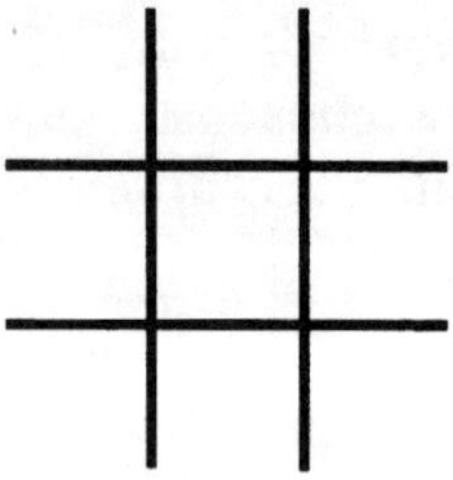

Schizoid

While We Wait for Designer Genes, We Have

Designer Drugs

David J. Robinson, M.D.

Haldol, the original "alldol"

Brawldol	Subdues aggressive tendencies
Calldol	Keeps the ward quiet when you're on call
Balldol	Reduces erotomanic fixations
Appalldol	Subdues indignation (even if unwarranted)
Falldol	Unique action raises blood pressure to counteract the lightheadedness that occurs with other medications
Smalldol	Pediatric preparation for psychotic infants
Crawldol	Stops delusional wandering in toddlers
Drawldol	Prevents speech from becoming slurred
Stalldol	Help for the terminally dyskinetic
Malldol	Decreases impulsivity in shopaholics
Galldol	Adds supreme confidence for stressful times
Y'alldol	Helps overcome anxiety when greeting strangers
Squalldol	Diminishes tempestuous outbursts

Television Previews:

Presenting the Anxiety Channel: Television Programming for the Fearful and Phobic

Your Announcer is Joel Kirschbaum, Ph.D.
Hillsborough, New Jersey

Starting script: Subscribe today for the series of books entitled, "Food Hazards." Begin with your free copy of "Calories Part A — 300 foods whose main ingredient consists of sugar fried in lard." You will then receive a volume detailing dangerous diets every month for the rest of your lengthened life.

In science news: Molecular biologists have disabled the genes in humans that cause aging. To ensure a secure retirement, you can now work for a newly discovered intergalactic civilization that needs zoological specimens. Criteria for "employment" are the ability to perform both acrobatics and usually private acts in public and willingness to nuzzle various beings with unfamiliar forms. The chosen human volunteers will receive free room and board, as well as any needed veterinary care. Fortunately, these extraterrestrials are vegans.

But now, a message: Did you try a sample copy of the magazine "Danger!"? This month's issue features the locations of the world's twenty most seismically stable locations. You'll be shocked by the expose "Expiration Dates — Great for the Gullible." You'll be pleased to see that all of the magazine's pages have rounded edges to prevent catastrophic paper cuts.

News flash: Another asteroid has been discovered with an orbit within less than a million miles of our defenseless planet. This now makes a total of two million celestial objects, any one of which might collide with us at any time — even if we're in our beds and under the covers.

And now, a question for you: Are you free of any odd aches, pains, or peculiar sensations? Then you'll want to buy the book "Send Me a Sign" which describes over 300 possible fatal diseases (including Ebola infection, brain tumors and dementia) that begin with no symptoms. The videotape version is made out of material strong enough to support a person. Once the tape is unwound from the cassette and safely anchored, it will permit you to safely escape quicksand, crumbling cliffs, and burning buildings. The DVD version is reflective so that if you become stranded you can use it to signal rescuers.

In the fashion news, you'll want your very own isolation suit, with a dedicated air-purifier after you read our booklets, "2001 Diseases Transmitted by Air or Touch" and "How to Avoid Hepatitis When the Virus Mutates And Becomes As Easy to Catch as the Common Cold." You'll want the optional helmet which can constantly transmit your location, by way of global positioning satellites, to immediately:

1. Notify agoraphobics of impending precipices
2. Provide proof, when falsely accused of a violent crime, that you were somewhere else via this "Instant Alibi," or
3. Send rescuers if you signal that you are either somewhere confusing, engulfed by an avalanche, or are overcome by amnesia.

Finally, a word about our late-night docudramas/infomercials. Watch for "Inspection Time" a do-it-yourself feature on how you can use mirrors, positioned on flexible, hinged rods, to inspect every square inch of your skin for any newly-developed imperfections that may require immediate medical attention. It is easy-to-adjust so you can check yourself every few hours at home, at work and (with an available spotlight accessory) even at movies, concerts or the theater. Coming next week, the docudrama "Intimations of Infidelity — Other People's Underwear Inside Out."

Final commercial: Do you work in a small, windowless office or cubicle? Do you ever feel like the walls contracting around you? Improve your mental health and morale by ordering a mural of outdoor scenery as viewed from the safety of ground level. Or, while seated at your desk, you can be surrounded by the image of you giving a stage fright free lecture at the *Institute for Advanced Study,* to a standing ovation by wildly applauding Nobel Laureates. These peel-off 8′ by 4′ decals will also bolster your self-esteem. They affix to all walls, and can easily be trimmed to expose the exit sign.

Signoff: This Station is part of the Enablers' Network.

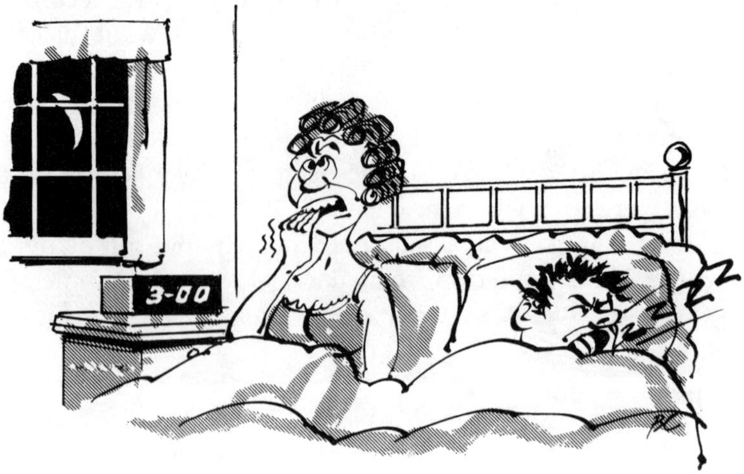

Rapid Psychler Cards

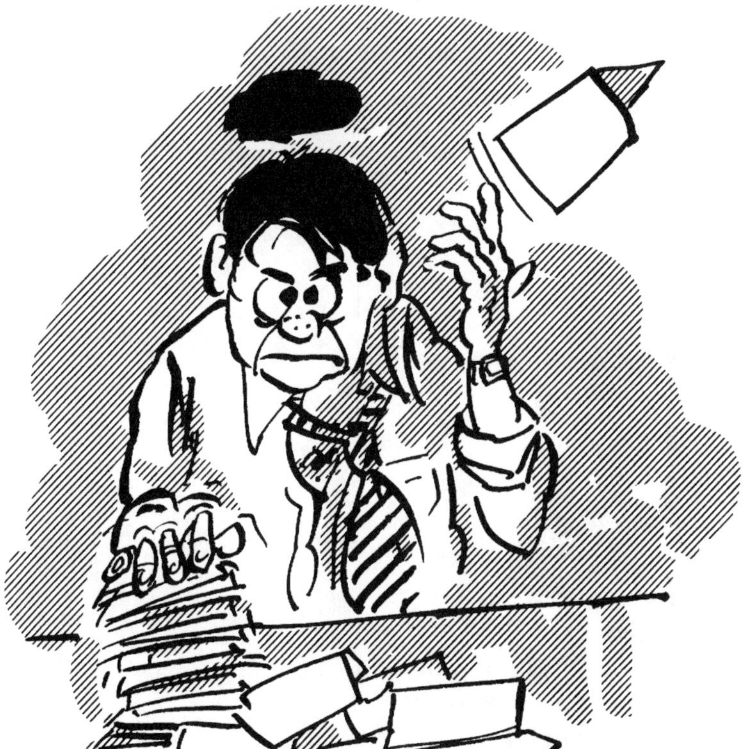

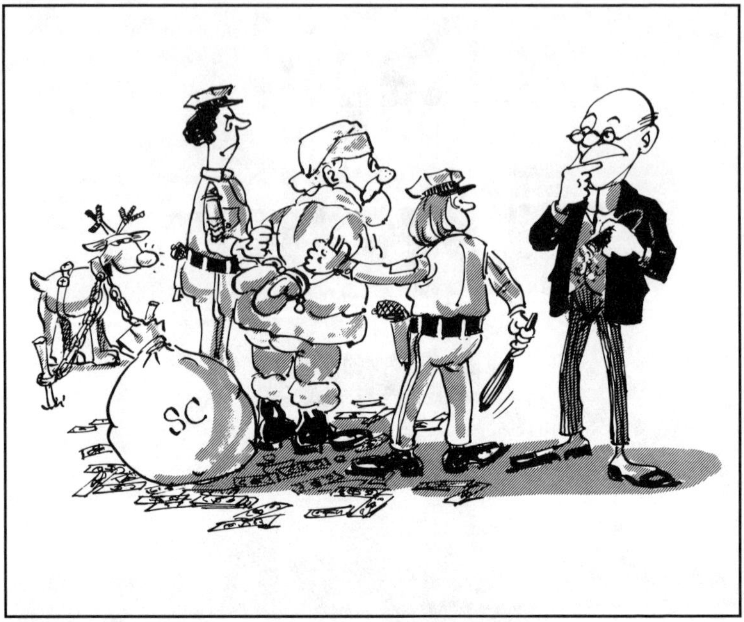

Inside Caption

"We arrested Mr. Claus for running an illegal workshop in Antarctica. He said he wanted to be *bipolar*."

Features
- Full color
- Portrait (upright) orientation
- Folded in packages of 10 with envelopes
- Shrink-wrapped
- $15.00 USD

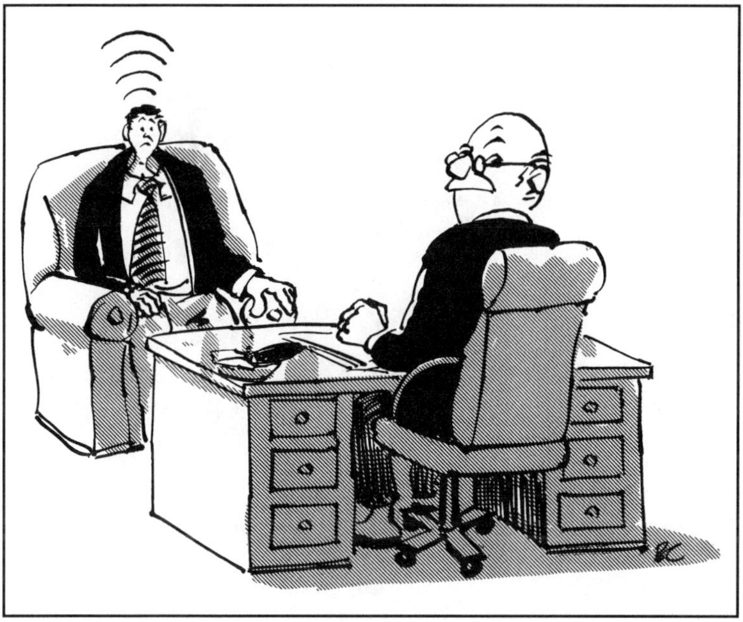

Inside Caption

"If you can't stay in sight, at least stay in touch."

Features

- Full color
- Portrait (upright) orientation
- Folded in packages of 10 with envelopes
- Shrink-wrapped
- $15.00 USD

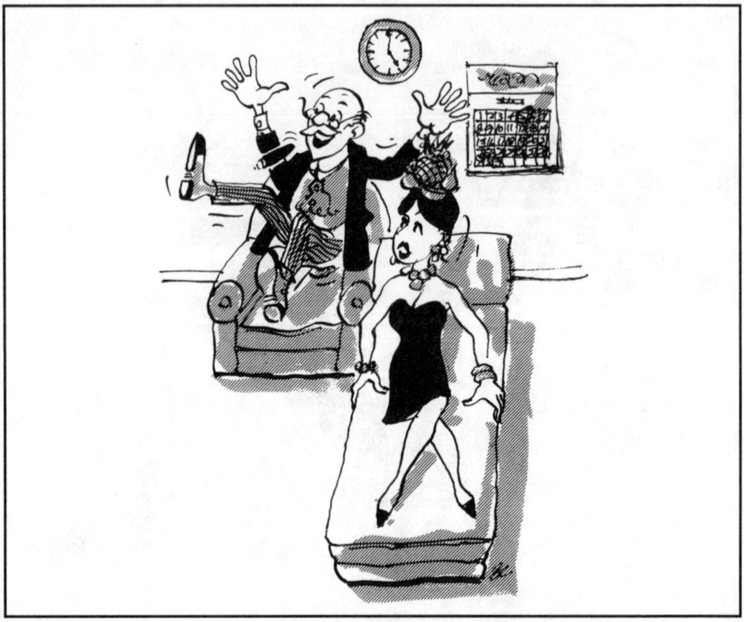

Inside Caption

"The holidays are coming.
Get hysterical."

Features
- Full color
- Portrait (upright) orientation
- Folded in packages of 10 with envelopes
- Shrink-wrapped
- $15.00 USD

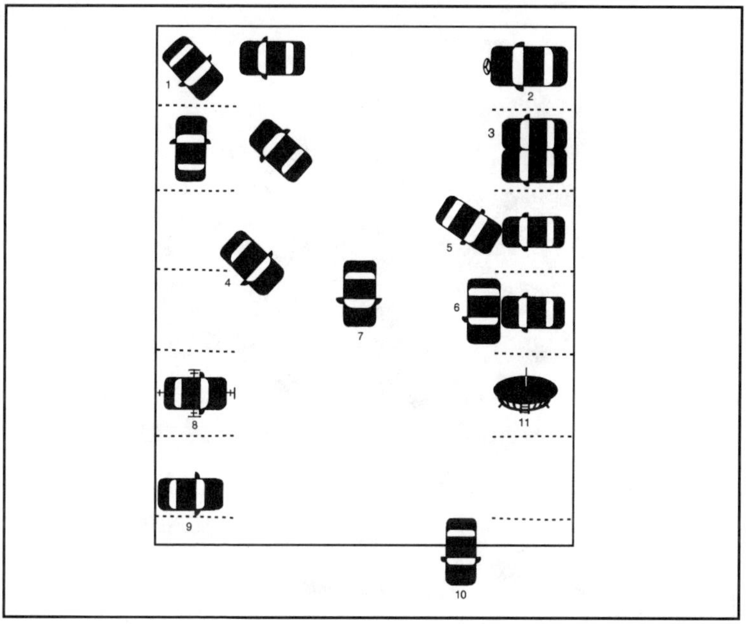

Inside Caption

1. Paranoid	Cornered again!!
2. Narcissist	Largest car; prominent hood ornament
3. Dependent	Needs other cars to feel sheltered
4. Passive-Aggressive	Angles car to take two spaces
5. Borderline	Rams into car of ex-lover
6. Antisocial	Obstructs other cars
7. Histrionic	Parks in center of lot for dramatic effect
8. Obsessive	Perfect alignment in parking spot
9. Avoidant	Hides in corner
10. Schizoid	Can't tolerate closeness to other cars
11. Schizotypal	Intergalactic parking

Features

- Full color
- Portrait (upright) orientation
- Folded in packages of 10 with envelopes
- Shrink-wrapped
- $15.00 USD

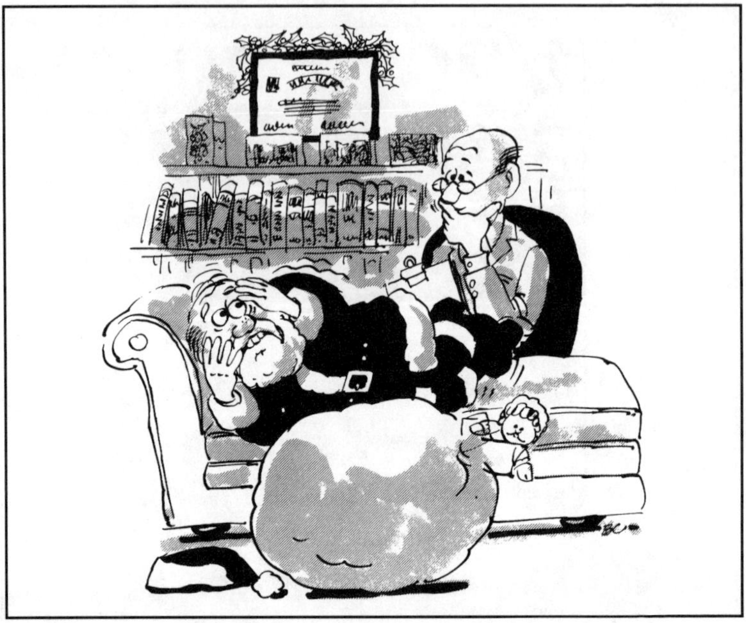

Inside Caption

"This is clearly a case of Santaclaustrophobia."

Features

- Full color
- Portrait (upright) orientation
- Folded in packages of 10 with envelopes
- Shrink-wrapped
- $15.00 USD